What on Earth Can I Eat?

Food, Type 2 Diabetes and

YOU

by

Alan Shanley

Everything in Moderation – Except Laughter

What on Earth Can I Eat?

First Edition published 2010

Alan Shanley, Pottsville, Australia

Copyright © Alan Shanley 2010

Printed in the United States of America.

1) Diabetes 2) Diet 3) Health 4) Self-Monitoring Blood Glucose

This book is based on the author's own experience and research as a type 2 diabetic and is not aimed to replace any advice you may receive from your medical practitioner. The publisher and author of this book assume no responsibility or liability whatsoever on the behalf of any purchaser or reader of these materials. The author is not a doctor, nor does he claim to be. No action should be taken based solely on the contents of this book. Readers should consult appropriate health professionals on any matter relating to their health and well being.

ISBN-13: 978-1453863213
ISBN-10: 1453863214

Acknowledgements

I am immensely grateful to all of the people who helped me so much on usenet's diabetes newsgroups misc.health.diabetes and alt.support.diabetes when I was a scared, brand new type 2 diabetic and also to the many people I have encountered since on the ADA forum, the dLife forum, the UK Diabetes Support forum and the diabetesworld Yahoo group.

I owe special thanks to my wife Lorraine, who has supplied love, understanding and innumerable cups of coffee for countless mornings as I left her for my virtual companions on a personal diabetes journey in cyberspace.

Appreciation from Readers

As this is the first edition of my first book the following comments are selected from responses on forums, personal emails or comments on my blog. I have edited for brevity, indicated by "..." but I have not changed any words. Only first names are provided for privacy reasons.

From the ADA Forum.

I have wanted to tell you for several months now how much reading your blog has helped me ... I had severe stomach pains, went to the ER - had acute pancreatitis caused by gallstones resulting in emergency gallbladder removal surgery. Oh, and by the way, you have diabetes. I was in the hospital for a week and they sent a nutritionist to see me.

Turns out she was the same one I had seen the week before when I was going to get lapband surgery. She gave me the food pyramid handout and told me to eat pretty much like they were finally feeding me in the hospital. Breakfast: french toast and high carb cereal. She also told me to go ahead with getting the surgery and it would take care of the diabetes.

I also saw an Endo who put me on lantus & novolog ... I really had no idea what to eat and really didn't have any hunger anyway ... At first I wasn't sure if you all were right because it wasn't what I learned in the hospital but I kept reading and also bought some of the recommended books. I educated myself with your help. I also have lost 85 lbs so far this year by going low carb. My a1c went from 9.2 in January to 5.8 in May. It was then, and only then that I cried. I feel great and my test results are great. I owe so much to you and I just wanted to send you this personal note to say THANK YOU SO VERY MUCH.

Gayle,

Alan, your's was one of the very first greetings I received at the ADA website about three years ago when I was officially diagnosed as "Diabetic" and turned out into the big, confusing world without enough guidance. Your blog was warm and humorous and EXTREMELY helpful. You addressed the basic issues in a straightforward way. I have learned so very much under your teaching. As you helped me understand, diabetes is a personal disease and what works for one person may not work for another. Your steady guiding back to "test, adjust, test" has been invaluable

Elisse

Your blog and contributions to the ADA forum inspired me to start researching diabetes and become both an advocate for my health and after seeing the results I got following your suggestions I have gotten active spreading the message. If only the CDE's would read what you have written, it would save toes!

Neil

Alan, your blog and precise instructions to me on the ADA board have been the basis for my trip to controlling my BG. Your forthright feedback has served me well and I wish that all the forums had a link to your blog. Many misconceptions I read on forums could be corrected!

Penny

From the Diabetes Support Forum UK.

I am one of the founders of Diabetes-support.org.uk forum and find Alan's site a never endingly useful place to point newly diagnosed diabetics where they can find excellent advice, tips for eating and other very down to earth and common sense information on diabetes. We use it as one of the resources to tack onto our own website. He has excellent knowledge of the condition and is an expert on T2 not to mention cholesterol issues.

Patti

Alan's advice has been signposted to fellow diabetics many times on this site - for good reason... I have a healthy respect for the disciplines of both science and medicine and Alan's advice manages to bridge the gap between the two in a way that allows you to see beyond the mainstream view but without having to have the analytical brain of a NASA scientist ... Although Alan is Type 2 ... Alan's advice will ... offer something for everyone. What's more, it's included with a wry look at the world, and a smile.

Lib, Type 1,

I can't wait for Alan's book. As someone involved with UK diabetes forums I know first-hand that good sensible unpatronising down-to-earth peer advice is invaluable. It is no understatement to say it saves lives. T2s face much conflicting and confusing information. ... I regularly recommended Alan's excellent blogs as a prime source of information, hope and inspiration. Based on extensive research, but delivered in an accessible non-judgemental way, they are a world-class resource. Little wonder, then, that Alan is trusted and admired across the globe.

Terry

From my blog: Type 2 Diabetes – A Personal Journey

Alan, you have been an invaluable resource for my husband, Bob, who was diagnosed with type two last fall. We were completely ignorant about diabetes. There had never been any in either of our families and my husband is not obese and never has been. Your suggestions have been his best and easiest to access resource.

Margie

Thank you, Alan, for your wonderfully readable, and very useful, tips for traveling with diabetes ...You've given me hope, and concrete tips, for resuming travel both by car and by air.

Heidi

When I was first diagnosed as a Type 2, your site was one of the first I found ... You have a real talent in distilling information and also conveying an upbeat "take control of your life" attitude. I would suspect you have no idea how many people you have helped.

Bob

Your words of advice have been kind, forthright, humorous and full of real-life information. I am SO grateful that you were there as a resource on the ADA boards from my very first "pre-diabetic" question. With your firm encouragement and the others on the board, I bought myself a glucose meter, used it almost painlessly from the beginning and knew just what to aim for as I adjusted my diet and life. Without your comments, I think I might have gone for years without making any significant changes in my lifestyle until it was almost too late. My doctor now says I am the most successful patient she has ever had at changing her life for the better, and you were really the one responsible for that.

Athena

I've been reading Alan's work on the web for more than 5 years and have been reading his blog in particular since it was started ... His writing is well-researched, clear and written in a personal style that makes it easily understandable and allows people to relate the subject to their own situation. Alan has helped hundreds of type 2 diabetics all over the world, some of whom he's not even aware of ... I don't hesitate to recommend his writing to any diabetic

Anonymous

Hi Alan. ... Wow! What an amazing info filled site! I've been Diabetic for 10 yrs, on Metformin for 8 yrs, on slow release insulin at night for 6 months. And never have I seen better information Thank you!

Bonita

I found your article on painless blood glucose monitor testing especially useful! By applying what I've read here and on Jenny Ruhl's Blood Glucose 101 site, I've gotten my a1c down to 5.3% (from 9.5% a year ago) and am feeling better than ever!

Julianne

I also have been using Alan's site as a primary source for newbies in the various newsgroups and forums I inhabit. It makes an easy to read and easy to use antidote to the often woeful "official" advice.

Chris

CONTENTS

INTRODUCTION

Chapter 1. Diabetes and Diet

Whether you have just been diagnosed with diabetes or you have been fighting this condition for many years the single most confusing question facing you as a type 2 diabetic is "what should I eat?"

We are bombarded with conflicting answers from all sides; from doctors, dieticians, diabetes educators, magazines, newspapers, TV, the internet, family and friends. They all claim to be right but many will be wrong.

This book is intended to help you answer that question – for you.

One of the problems with all of those conflicting sources of dietary advice is that they are generalised. The people promoting the conflicting and confusing array of diets, herbal cures, supplements and other magic bullets do not know you as well as you do. Nor do they know your other medical conditions, your food allergies, your exercise limitations or how your body reacts to different foods at different times of the day.

My intention is to show you how to find a way of eating that suits you, and you alone, to help control blood glucose levels, achieve and maintain optimum weight, provide good nutrition and minimise the possibility of future complications from diabetes.

New to diabetes?

Are you newly diagnosed? Possibly you have just found out you have type 2 diabetes? Or impaired glucose tolerance? Or impaired fasting glucose? Or pre-diabetes? Or the doctor said "you have got a touch of sugar" or something similar?

And you're in shock?

Why me?

Well, I do not really have an answer for that. To me it seemed bloody unfair. Why me? What did I do to deserve this? And I railed against the world for a while. But then I decided to get on with it. Because I cannot change the past and how can I correct the mistake of choosing the wrong grandparents? Particularly as I liked mine.

What about the old-timers?

Or maybe you have had diabetes for many years. You initially tried to do all the things your doctors and dieticians told you would help. You took your medications and you "ate healthy" and you did some exercise and you tried hard.

It worked for a little while. You lost some weight, maybe a lot of weight. Your HbA1c and fasting numbers got better.

But then it stopped working so well and it got harder to stick to the diet and you lost fitness, gained weight, added more medications or insulin and lost that initial drive to beat this condition. Now the doctor looks gloomy and says that you will inevitably progress to those nasty complications unless you change. But you do not know what is left to change or how to do it and you are nervous about adding extra medications. Or maybe those complications are already appearing. So you keep asking yourself – what now?

The blame game

My first suggestion is the most important one of all. It is **NOT** your fault. Take a deep breath, sit back, and relax.

Forget the hype and the TV ads about obesity, lifestyle, whatever - that is in the past, even if it was relevant, and there is not a darn thing you can do about it. Those TV ads do not mention that 10-15% of type 2 diabetics are normal weight or underweight at diagnosis. I wasn't slim so I will talk about the rest of us and how to lose that excess weight later in this book.

You should also forget everything you think you know about "eating healthy". Start again with a clean slate, because a lot of the things the dieticians told us in the 20th century are slowly being proved to be wrong in the 21st.

Now is the time to act

OK. So you have a flawed glucose/insulin system. I do not care what label they put on it, or what stage you are at, what matters is what you intend to do about it. First, the good news. Unless you have been diagnosed at a very late stage, this is a slow-moving disease. You have time to learn, time to correct things and time to improve your health for a long-term future. There is more good news. Nearly every person I know who used this diagnosis as a kick-start to get fitter and healthier has improved many other aspects of their health at the same time.

I wrote this book for all type 2 diabetics; but, to be honest, I know it is not really for everyone. If you are one of the vast majority of type 2 diabetics who are content to let their doctor manage their condition by taking the prescribed pills or insulin and doing little else, then stop now.

If your idea of watching your diet is to order diet coke with the Big Mac meal; or ordering steamed brown rice instead of fried rice with your Chinese dinner; or whole wheat instead of white bread for your lunch sandwich then I probably can't help you. I have a diabetic friend who claims his main form of exercise is jumping to conclusions or sweeping the room with a glance. This is not for him either.

I wrote this book for the many people with type 2 diabetes who are prepared to do a little extra to save their lives or improve their health. I can offer big rewards in terms of health for that small extra effort, but only if you do the work.

That does not mean that I will be telling you to train for the Olympics, or even to run around the block; but I will be suggesting some moderate exercise. Nor does it mean that I will be suggesting an extreme diet, eating cardboard bread and plastic cheese with rabbit food; but I will be showing you how to make some effective improvements to your present way of eating.

Are you prepared to do a bit extra, with the possibility of living a longer, happier life by deferring or delaying the terrible complications of diabetes? I hope so. My own goal is for those complications to arrive about ten years after I depart the planet in my sleep as a very old man.

The scope of this book

I should make it clear what this book is about, and also what it is not about.

My primary purpose is to help individual type 2 diabetics develop a lifestyle that is enjoyable and sustainable but which is also effective in achieving and maintaining good blood glucose control, good weight management and good nutrition. The methods I concentrate on are dietary change, home blood glucose testing, moderate exercise and other lifestyle aspects.

This book is not about medications or insulin. Although I may occasionally mention insulin and oral medications, I do not offer any medical advice and do not offer any suggestions on medication or insulin prescription, doses, or suitability. Any questions on medications or insulin should be answered by your doctor or diabetes educator who will have a full knowledge of your personal situation.

As this book is written as a result of my personal journey with type 2 diabetes it may help if I describe some of that journey.

There are turning points in all our lives. Some we only recognise in hindsight, while others are immediately obvious.

D-day No. 1

D is for diagnosis. My life changed completely four days before my 55th birthday in February 2002. Our village had a local doctor for the first time in several years. A couple of years before that the doctor I travelled to see in the city had told me "your cholesterol is a little high, but you do not need to worry - we have a pill that fixes that." He prescribed a statin, Lipitor 20mg. He never mentioned my 120Kg (260lbs) weight, or my fasting blood glucose levels of 7.9mmol/L (140mg/dL), or diet, or exercise, or even the hint of diabetes. Just an instruction to "take this pill." So I took the pill, and changed nothing else. I was fat and happy. Does that sound familiar to anyone?

The new doctor was a much wiser doctor than the one I used to see in the city. Instead of just renewing the statin prescription he said that he needed to see me first. He impressed me at that appointment by painlessly filling several different pathology bottles with samples of my blood. Little did I realise how much those samples were going to change my life. A few days later I received a call from his receptionist asking me to see the doctor to discuss my blood tests.

On the day my life changed I sat in the doctor's office and went into shock as he told me I had leukaemia. You thought I was going to say Type 2 Diabetes, didn't you? No – on that day in February 2002 he told me I had Chronic Lymphocytic Leukaemia, CLL. Happy birthday...

I went home in a daze. I was semi-retired at the time. By the time I reached home, I had made up my mind to be "officially" retired and that I was going to do some of the things I had always wanted to do. I was not going to die with my song unsung. So when I returned home I told my wife as she opened the door that I was going to travel around the world. I had always wanted to travel but always spent the time or money on something more important or more responsible. It was only later in the day I got up the courage to tell her why. A year later we went around the world for the first time. Incidentally, if you're interested in travel, I have blogged about my trips here: http://loraltravel.blogspot.com, "Born Under A Wandering Star".

Over the next two months I went through all the fun things of confirming my cancer diagnosis; a multitude of blood tests and a bone marrow aspiration. Ouch. I got on the Web and searched for things I could do to help myself beat it. I found nothing. Zero. Zip. Nada.

The depression of diagnosis set in. I was told I was on "W&W", watch and wait. Wrong. "W&W" really means wonder and worry.

D-day No. 2

And then, just two months later in April 2002 my doctor told me I also had Type 2 diabetes. Those earlier blood tests had led to him following up with an HbA1c test. The result was 8.2%.

Oh joy.

But this was different. He advised me to lose 8% of my body-weight and to get a blood glucose test meter. He suggested I test fasting and pre-dinner blood glucose levels and gave me targets for these numbers. He gave me several pamphlets on diet, mostly from Diabetes Australia. Unfortunately those did not help much with practical advice on how to achieve those blood glucose targets. He also asked if I wanted to see a dietician; in my ignorance I said no. Later, when I had learned a little more, I changed that decision.

The CLL diagnosis had primed me. There I was, frustrated and depressed because of my impotence in dealing with the CLL; now suddenly I had a goal that I could work towards.

Weight Loss

I hit the ground running. I designed my own weight-loss cooking and eating plan and put it into practice. You will find it at Chapter 8. And it worked. When I lost the 8%, I just kept going until I eventually lost over 20% of my body weight. It isn't rocket science, but it does take some self-discipline.

I had assumed that losing the weight would fix the problem and my diabetes would go away. But it was not enough and it did not go away. My HbA1c only dropped from 8.2% to 7.5%, despite my weight loss. I also continued to see alarming numbers when I tested randomly after meals, but I had no idea how to change that.

Searching for answers

I was thirsty for more information. Over the next couple of months I attended personal dietician's consultations and a local dietician's diabetes education course. They all had the same advice: eat a balanced diet. Their definition of balanced was to avoid all forms of fat like the plague and to eat lots of vegetables, lots of fruit and lots of whole grains; especially at breakfast.

My weight loss stalled and my blood glucose levels got worse as I started adding extra carbohydrates to follow the dietician's advice. I learned a lot from the dieticians, because before that I did not even know what a carbohydrate was, but the low fat, high whole grains advice was disastrous for me when I put it into practice.

Discovery

Then, like a new world, I discovered the anarchy of usenet's diabetes groups and eventually the most powerful, simple, logical advice I have seen before or since for new type 2 diabetics.

That original advice is written by a lady with type 2 diabetes named Jennifer. You will find a copy of it at Appendix C. In essence, she says to test after you eat to see what your food does to you. Then change what you eat to improve the results next time. That is basically it. So simple, but so incredibly effective and powerful if you think about it and then put it into practice. Naturally, everyone who uses it adapts it for themselves and over time I modified it for my own use as described in Chapter 6, Testing, Testing.

It is simplistic to concentrate only on blood glucose levels and I reviewed other aspects of nutrition periodically as I made those changes. But I always made blood glucose control the first priority.

Since I received that double diagnosis I have spent almost every morning, when I was not travelling, in front of the computer reading and writing to other people with diabetes on the net and the web in many different forums. I list some of those forums in

Appendix E, Books and Links. I turned my affliction into my hobby. I learned to use the various medical search engines on the web and subscribed to email alerts from sites such as the New England Journal of Medicine, the American Diabetes Association, Journal of the American Medical Association, Heart, Endocrine Today, Diabetes in Control and many others. I read everything I could find. I learned to understand "Medi-speak" and how to pick a valid research paper from a poor one; and believe me, there are far too many poor ones. Some of those papers I understood, some I got others to explain to me, and some of their ideas I put into practice using Jennifer's closing advice of "use your body as a science experiment".

Within the first year, using only testing, diet and exercise I had lost over 20% of my body weight, reduced my HbA1c to near 6% (under 6% shortly afterwards) and reduced fasting blood glucose levels to under 6mmol/L (108mg/dL). Those are my continuing primary targets.

Will this work for you?

I am just one person with type 2 diabetes, a condition which is slightly different for every single one of us. What works for me may not work for you. So, why should I think that it may?

I learned a lot from many good people on the usenet groups and over time I started trying to help others as they arrived, shocked and scared, on those forums. If their situation sounded like mine and I felt I could suggest a way to help, I did. And slowly, over time, I found that many people started to experiment for themselves using my suggestions and they worked for them too. Often we both learned from the mutual feedback of advice and experiment.

Over time I found that I am a good coach. Like many coaches, I found that some of those I helped achieved better results than the coach. I respect them but I do not envy them, because we each have to choose the right balance for ourselves. I could work harder and achieve tighter goals, but I balance that with my enjoyment of life. My signature on the web is "Everything in Moderation – Except Laughter". I keep that in mind when making lifestyle decisions. But I never forget that the laughter may become a bit strained if the terrible diabetes complications start to appear in my life. So I try to make sure I work just hard enough to ensure they do not. That can never be guaranteed – but after more than eight years they have not arrived yet.

After a while I added other forums and groups to my morning and the number of new arrivals I responded to started to grow, especially on the American Diabetes Association (ADA) Forum. I found that I was repeating myself daily. So I looked for a way to store the "standard" suggestions and discovered blogging. My blog started in 2006 as a type of archive, a way to give a new person a link to more information without typing it several times daily. Then it started to grow, as I answered more questions and posted some of those answers to the blog.

This book grew out of that experience, partly to help those who are more comfortable with a book than a computer screen. I finally made the decision to write this book when many of those who had followed my suggestions over the years urged me to write it.

A fortunate accident

Serendipity is a wonderful thing. These days I spend a lot of my time on various web and net diabetes forums trying to persuade newly diagnosed or poorly controlled type 2 diabetics to use after-meal testing to adjust their way of eating. I am out-spoken on the effects of diet on diabetes. However, I make no claims about diet and leukaemia. But something odd happened. My CLL numbers all improved as I took control of my diet for diabetes.

For several years I was involved in the excellent ACOR mailing list for support and information for CLL, eventually becoming one of the list managers. If you are interested in that list or the other ACOR cancer support lists you will find them at www.acor.org. My improvement eventually led to me resigning from the CLL list. It became increasingly difficult to see old friends passing away or in pain as I improved. If the Sword of Damocles drops and the numbers start rising again I will return, but for now I just see the haematologist annually and get on with the rest of my life.

My haematologists remind me that it is serendipitous, but they also tell me to keep doing what I am doing. That sounds like good advice to me, so I will.

Location, location

I am an Australian and I wrote this book from a very personal viewpoint. As a consequence readers from the USA will quickly notice I spell words oddly at times and approach things from a slightly different slant. For diabetes we add another source of possible confusion: we use different numbers for blood glucose levels.

For that reason I have tried to minimise (not minimize – don't worry about it) the use of numbers in the text and where they must appear I have used both terms. For example, in Chapter 5, Exercise, I write "If you often see high blood glucose levels of more than 250 mg/dL or 14 mmol/L you should test before commencing exercise." Do not let the different numbers confuse you; those two are almost identical blood glucose levels. Focus on numbers that are relevant to your location and ignore those that are not.

I clarify that subject in more detail in Appendix D, Millimoles and Milligrams.

Chapter 3. Choosing Wisely

One of the most difficult things about the treatment of incurable conditions such as type 2 diabetes is the variety of advice available to us. Everyone has an opinion. In addition to advice from our doctors and diabetes educators advice is offered, whether we want it or not, from every quarter including television, magazines, newspapers, books, relatives, friends and colleagues. Unfortunately, much of it is bad or ignorant advice. So, we should only listen to the experts, right?

The answer is a definite maybe.

Even the experts and the major diabetes authorities disagree over treatment, medications, diet and the right blood glucose targets to aim for. Sometimes the differences are trivial, but at other times they can be very significant. It gets even more confusing when you read of the differences between those authorities and the pro-active patients out there in the real world struggling to beat diabetes, each in our own way.

In the years since I was diagnosed with diabetes I have asked many experts many questions. Most gave excellent answers. But some did not answer at all; some, like politicians, ignored my questions and only gave answers to the questions I hadn't asked but that they wanted to answer; and some gave me answers that were more like orders and made my condition worse. Most of the latter group were dieticians.

Asking experts for advice is a very wise thing to do. Believing experts as though they are infallible and always know all the answers is not. To learn in any field, ask many experts, not one. When you do that you will find confusion because they won't all agree. It is up to you to read and learn enough to be able to assess the worth of their advice and decide which expert's advice to trust and which to discard. Ask the experts, but always pass all their advice through the filter of your own common sense. Remember that not all experts have letters after their name. Experience and expertise can make an expert. Examples that come to mind are Gretchen Becker, a "Patient Expert" who I learned a lot from myself; David Mendosa, who writes about diabetes on the web; or Jenny Ruhl, the author of Blood Sugar 101. I have also learned a lot from other diabetics on web forums who have "been there, done that". Even when they did it wrong, I learned from their reported mistakes.

When deciding who to listen to and who to ignore, never forget that the person who will be most affected by poor advice from any source will be you. Not me, not your doctor, not your dietician, but you. In my opinion, more than almost any other condition, the success of management of diabetes depends on the diabetic. Although your medics can advise and prescribe, it is your decisions and your actions that will decide your future.

TAKING CONTROL

This is an over-view of the plan for your own action in addition to anything the doctors prescribe. A more detailed expansion of each suggestion will be found in the later chapters mentioned here.

What to Eat at First

You will have probably received some diet sheets from your doctor or a dietician. Some, a rare minority, are good. Most are not. It is still useful to read them, because they will include some valuable information but most will unfortunately recommend a diet that is low in fats and high in carbohydrates such as whole grains and fruits. Very few people can stick to those diets and even fewer succeed in managing good blood glucose levels using them. You will soon be using your meter and will quickly understand why I write that, but until then please read Appendix A, What to Eat at First, to help you get through the first few days until you get organised.

Blood Glucose testing

If you do not have a blood glucose meter, obtain one. I cannot emphasise enough how important that is. Your meter will become your single most effective weapon in your war on diabetes and its complications.

Learn how to test your blood glucose levels. If you are

worried about the idea of poking holes in yourself see Appendix B, Painless Pricks, to help you get started.

Use those tests to adjust your menu to improve your blood glucose numbers until they are approaching the non-diabetic range. Details on how to do that are in chapter 6, Testing, Testing.

Weight Loss

If you are overweight – lose it. No excuses. I have written some ideas on what I did to achieve that myself in Chapter 8, Weight Loss Cooking and Eating Plan.

If that does not suit you, then do whatever would work for you. However, be rather cautious about commercial plans and programmes that emphasise low fat methods. Such methods almost always have menus with a high carbohydrate content which are unlikely to be effective for you as a type 2 diabetic. You may lose weight in the short term but almost certainly your blood glucose levels will not be helped very much as a result and you will eventually regain that lost weight. If you must use a commercial plan I suggest Atkins or South Beach, but even those still need to be tested, using your meter, to adjust the menu to suit your unique needs.

Excessive weight is associated with increased insulin resistance and that will interfere with your efforts to manage blood glucose levels. Weight loss, if you are overweight, will assist in blood glucose control but it is not the total solution nor will it cure your diabetes. Obesity can also cause or exacerbate other significant health problems.

Exercise

Exercise is a vital part of diabetes management.

If you are one of those people who make me feel tired just to look at them as they jog purposefully past every morning, great, but I am not one of you. My ankles, which turn painfully but too easily, decreed many years ago that jogging is not for me. Instead I do "lazy man's exercise". Like Goldilocks: not too little, not too much, but just right – for me. In winter I walk down the street, or ride my bike around the neighbourhood for about a half-hour, or mow the lawns, or spend some time on my air-walker if the weather is bad. In summer I add a half-hour of freestyle in the pool to the mix.

You do not have to do anything extreme. Extreme exercise can cause injuries, which is a bit counter-productive to long term health in my opinion. You are not competing for a million dollars on the Biggest Loser, you are aiming to get a prize much greater than that: a healthier, happier, longer life.

I have given some tips on finding forms of exercise to suit you and your circumstances in the next chapter.

Review

Later, as your changes to your lifestyle for optimum weight and optimum blood glucose levels start to work, review your way of eating and adjust it to ensure you are not missing anything vital. Good nutrition requires more than just foods that do not raise your blood glucose levels. I found that a good way to achieve that without getting too complicated is to include as wide a variety as possible of foods, especially of meats, fish and vegetables. That also helps keep the menu interesting.

There is more to come but that is enough to start with. So stop reading, go and have a glass of wine or a diet soda, and think about something else for a while before continuing to the next chapter.

Chapter 5. Exercise

My main focus is to help you discover a better way of eating to help manage your diabetes, but it would be remiss of me not to mention that the other half of "diet and exercise" should not be ignored. I am not an exercise fanatic. I call my own efforts "lazy man's exercise" and I have to force myself to do it some days. But I know that it is both essential and beneficial. Not only does exercise have an immediate effect on blood glucose levels after meals, it also improves muscle tone which has an effect on reducing insulin resistance for longer-term benefits.

Add at least half an hour of moderate exercise to your day. That is a minimum, not a maximum. If that is a new activity for you, start easy and work up slowly – but do it. Tailor your exercise to suit you. Your choice will be affected by many things, from your ability to walk, swim or run to the nature of your neighbourhood.

In the other chapters in this book I offer suggestions to help you find a way of eating that not only assists in management of your blood glucose levels but that you can also comfortably enjoy for the rest of your life. Exercise is similar. You need to find a form of exercise that you can continue to do for the rest of your life; otherwise you will cease doing it.

Find what works for you within your physical, financial and environmental restrictions. That may appear to be a difficult task, but it is not optional. Find something you can do and start doing it. For those of us with type 2 diabetes the glib saying "use it or lose it" can become all too real when discussing our limbs.

The following ideas are just that. Ideas to make you think outside the square and consider what may suit you.

Exercise ideas

If your neighbourhood is suitable and your body is able, go for a daily walk. If weather or security makes your neighbourhood unsuitable for walking, consider buying a treadmill or an air-walker.

If you have access to a pool, swim. Swimming is a marvellous exercise because it uses all your muscles, promotes good breathing habits and does not stress your joints. If you do not have a pool, then consider becoming a member at a local pool or joining a gym that has one.

Walk to the shops if they are close enough and carry your groceries home or trundle them in a trolley. If it is too far to walk, make a habit of parking further from the main door of the shopping mall instead of trying to park as near as possible.

If the weather is too hot or too cold for a walk, remember that your local shopping mall is usually air-conditioned and probably has plenty of room for a continuous half-hour walk. You will probably meet other "mall-walkers" there once you start.

If you live or work in a multi-story building, use the stairs instead of the lift or elevator to get to nearby floors.

Buy a bicycle if you can ride one safely in your district. I found that I was rather shaky the first time I got back on a bike after a twenty-five year gap. But the old saying is true – you never forget how to ride one. Just take care in the traffic. You do not want to end up as the fittest diabetic ever run over by a bus.

Make that extra effort and you will be surprised how much it helps your long-term blood glucose control. You can do more if you want to, but try to do at least half an hour a day.

If you are wheel-chair-bound or bed-bound, there are still exercises you can do, even if all you can move is your arms. Think outside the square. Move what you can, when you can, any way you safely can. There are also lots of web-sites to help you. Do some searches on "chair dancing" or "wheel-chair exercises" and similar terms.

I found that it helped minimise my after-meal blood glucose spikes if I timed the exercise to be not too long after meals.

A word of warning on exercise

If you often see high blood glucose levels of more than 250 mg/dL or 14 mmol/L you should test before commencing exercise. Arduous exercise at those levels may actually make high blood glucose levels worse.

In those circumstances you should discuss the suitability of exercise with your doctor before doing anything strenuous. If you decide to exercise after seeing a high reading, then test again during the exercise. If your blood glucose levels are rising instead of falling then cease that exercise and wait for a time when your numbers are better.

But If I Lose weight, I am Cured, Right?

Wrong. You will just be a slimmer, fitter type 2 diabetic.

In Chapter 8, Weight Loss Cooking and Eating Plan, I mention that when I was first diagnosed the doctor told me to lose 8% of my body weight and to test my blood glucose before breakfast and before the evening meal. I weighed 117Kg or 257lbs at that time; 8% of 117Kg is 9.4Kg or a little over 20lbs. My HbA1c was 8.2%.

Using my plan I achieved that weight loss and decided to keep going after I passed the 8% point.

I was disappointed to find that my HbA1c only dropped to 7.5% despite losing the weight. Consequently, I decided that the time had come to attend a dietician's presentation at a local diabetes support group meeting. Later, I also attended a group course with that dietician and had personal consultations with a couple of other dieticians. They all promoted the high carbohydrate, low fat, dietary guidelines issued at that time by Diabetes Australia and the American Diabetes Association.

Low Carb, High Carb and All That

At this point I should define some terms because "low fat", "high carb" and "low carb" seem to have different meanings for different people. I do not define my own way of eating that way, but others may.

I still have my notes from that course and some brochures I received from my doctor on diagnosis day. In brief, the emphasis was all on cutting calories and fat and eating plenty of grains and fruits. Little mention was made of the effects of high-carbohydrate meals on blood glucose but a great deal of importance was placed on the need to eat a minimum level of carbohydrates each day. They also re-defined the word "carb" to be 15 gms of carbohydrate, based on the out-dated Exchange Diet from last century.

The minimum recommended carbohydrate portion for each meal was two "carbs" for women and three "carbs" for men, with at least three one "carb" snacks over the course of a day. It was suggested that a little higher than that was better. Consequently, the daily total male and female recommendations were 12-15 and 9-12 "carbs" respectively. Translated to grams that is a minimum recommendation of 180-225 gms of carbohydrate daily for men and 135-180 gms for women. That is a lot lower in carbohydrates than the Standard American Diet or SAD (what a beautifully descriptive acronym), so in theory it could be called low-carbohydrate. However, compared to what I eat now it is high in carbohydrates.

I was not taught a minimum level for fats and oils, beyond a general impression that all fats are evil and should be avoided like the bubonic plague. I vaguely recall that there was a grudging acceptance, in answer to a question from the audience during a dietician's presentation, that some fats are OK and that it is acceptable to use olive oil on your salad, but sparingly.

I attempted to follow that advice. After all, these were the experts. Consequently, I made changes to my successful weight-loss menu in accordance with their teaching. Late in the course I coincidentally discovered the technique of testing after meals and I was shocked to see that the high carbohydrate, low fat guidelines were an absolute disaster for my blood glucose levels.

The Low Spike Way of Eating

There are interminable arguments these days about "low fat" versus "low carb". To be honest I am not interested in those definitions. What I was looking for was the "low blood glucose spike, excellent nutrition" menu that suited me. As to the "low blood glucose spike, excellent nutrition" menu that will suit you, you will have to test to find your own. Here is how I did that.

While doing the course with the dietician I found

misc.health.diabetes on usenet and eventually I was directed to Jennifer's wonderful "Test, test, test" advice. You will find it in Appendix C. Jennifer is not a doctor either, just another type 2 diabetic. But that advice works and it is free to all. I owe a great debt of thanks to Jennifer. Reading that web-page changed my life. She has graciously given permission for me to repeat her article in this book.

I started following her advice and the results, in a very short time, were quite dramatic. My fasting blood glucose and A1c started going down, my after-meal (called post-prandial by the medical people) numbers dropped rapidly, the occasions when I suffered "lows" with the shakes and nausea a couple of hours after meals almost disappeared and my weight loss re-commenced after being stalled for a few weeks.

The Effectiveness of Feedback from Testing

One of the reasons that testing after meals works so well is that it allows us to discover what works for us as individuals – and also what does not.

There are many tools out there to help us calculate the carbohydrate content of the foods we eat. They include web-sites, product labels, USDA nutrition tables and various software tools to analyse meals. They all have their uses, but none can predict exactly what the results will be in your body after you eat a meal.

On the other hand, your meter can be used to show exactly what the effect is. If you use it at the time of your blood glucose peak after a meal or snack you can then review the meal to assess what can be changed next time for a better result. If you do that enough times eventually the results will become very predictable, but only for you. I may get similar results, or I may not. The same applies to your friends and relatives with Type 2 diabetes; especially those who are always ready to tell you "of course you can eat that" at festive occasions or family functions, or worse, act as the Food Police and loudly proclaim to the assembled multitude that you must not eat a particular food.

Consider the complexity of diabetes. Each person, when first diagnosed with type 2 diabetes, has one or more flaws in their glucose/insulin system. They may have varying levels of insulin resistance, beta cell loss, signalling pathway faults for insulin or glycogen release or both, liver or kidney problems or digestive problems just to name a few. They may also have other associated or separate medical conditions. Add a few varied pills and supplements to the mix and then add varying levels of physical fitness and daily activity. On top of all that the new diabetic adds personal food allergies, likes and dislikes or ethnic or religious dietary restrictions.

When you think of it in those terms it is quite astounding that anyone could think that there are general dietary rules that could apply equally to all type 2 diabetics. That is why, in my opinion, the dietary guidelines put out by the various dietary and diabetes authorities are dangerously flawed. They make little allowance for individual variations. I have developed some basic guidelines of my own for brand new type 2 diabetics, see Appendix A, but those are a starting point, not an end point.

Your meter, if used correctly, will help guide you to the optimum way of eating for you based initially on your own likes, dislikes, allergies and restrictions.

Test timing

Most doctors or diabetes educators, if they recommend home testing at all, usually advise patients to test twice daily: before breakfast, also known as "fasting" and before the evening meal. Some, not many, also advise patients to test occasionally two hours after meals.

I have yet to meet a single newly diagnosed diabetic who was told by their doctor to find the timing of their blood glucose peak after meals and to test at that time.

So, why do I recommend that we should?

Any test is wasted if it neither informs nor confirms some information. The tests prescribed by your medical advisors are designed to help them analyse your progress to assist in their decisions for your treatment, usually to add more medications or insulin, but they do very little to help you personally manage your diabetes. The doctor wants to see your static or resting numbers; not the numbers that may be very high or even low as a result of the carbohydrates you ate or did not eat at your last meal.

That is why I use peak post-prandial tests; for simplicity I call them peak post-meal tests in this book. They help me directly. They are the dynamic numbers that show the direct effect of the food I eat and the exercise I do. In the early period after diagnosis that peak was more often a spike which is why I refer to this method as the low spike way of eating. The aim is to turn your spikes into gentle bumps.

Your peak will be slightly different but reasonably predictable with different foods and meal mixtures. Sweet drinks such as fruit juice or sugared sodas spike me very quickly within 30 minutes and drop just as quickly, which is why some people use them as a treatment for hypoglycaemia (low blood sugar) events. Starchy or sugary carbohydrates, without much fat, will spike me in 30-45 minutes. Add fat to those carbohydrates and my spike moves out to about 60 minutes. A normal meal combining moderate fat, moderate protein and moderate carbohydrates leads to a peak at 45-75 minutes for me. That is why I settled on using the one hour after-meal test as my guide, but I occasionally do a 30 minute test if the food was low in fats and high in carbohydrates.

Although my peak is about one hour after the last bite of my meal, yours may be different. Do some extra tests after meals to find out when your own peak occurs. Jennifer's advice solved the problem by recommending two tests after meals, at one hour and two hours. That works fine in the short term but can get a bit expensive for test strips and most people find such an intensive routine difficult to keep up for very long.

In the long run it is more effective and cheaper to discover your peak timing and stick to that. The best advice I have seen to help you find your own peak was written recently by Dr Lois Jovanovic, who is not only a top diabetes specialist but also a type 1 diabetic. Dr Jovanovic graciously granted me approval to include this quote from her advice to doctors in:

Using Meal-Based Self-Monitoring Blood Glucose (SMBG) Data to Guide Dietary Recommendations in Patients With Diabetes

The Diabetes Educator November 2009 vol. 35 no. 6 1023-1030

•• *Have patients determine the best time for postprandial SMBG by testing 45, 60, 75, 90, 105, and 120 minutes after a meal to detect their peak postprandial glucose concentration.*

I can't improve on that advice.

Test, Review, Adjust

This is the heart of my method. To summarise, it is as simple as this.

Discover your peak after-meal blood glucose spike time.

Eat, and then test after eating at your peak time. If blood glucose levels are too high then review what you ate and change the menu next time. Then do that again, and again, and again until what you eat does not spike your blood glucose levels.

You will get some surprises, particularly at breakfast time. The so-called "heart-healthy" breakfasts of cereal, milk, juice and fruit are NOT for most type 2 diabetics. Similarly, you will find variations through the day; the same foods may have different effects at breakfast, lunch, dinner and supper. But I can't say how they will affect others - only how it affected me - which is why you need to test yourself.

Then test again.

Test, review, adjust; always towards better and better blood glucose levels.

Too Much Testing?

I know that seems like a lot of testing; I agree that it is at first. But you won't have to test so intensively for the rest of your life. I always test with a purpose, to either learn or confirm knowledge. When I first read the "test, test, test" advice I put it into practice - totally. For a short period I tested before every meal and snack, then at one hour after the last bite and then at two hours. Of course, I was still learning at that time and I do not suggest that you need to do that; on some days I tested over 20 times. That period also taught me how to test painlessly as I describe in Appendix B, Painless Pricks.

Very quickly I found that some tests became very predictable. I soon dropped my pre-meal tests as unnecessary when I could predict them with good accuracy. Then, as I discovered that my own peak after-meal timing is one hour after I finish eating, I dropped the two-hour tests unless the one-hour result was unusual. Within a couple of weeks I was testing my pre-breakfast fasting level and my peak after-meal blood glucose level after every meal or snack, usually 5 to 8 times daily.

In a reasonably short time those tests became predictable too, as I slowly modified my diet from disastrous, as taught to me by the dieticians, to low spike. Within a few months I was testing from one to four times daily.

I test a lot less now that my personal data base of food blood glucose effects is fairly comprehensive. Usually I only test for maintenance to check that things have not changed. For several days I may not test at all, on other days I may test three or four times if trying a new recipe or menu.

I was learning as I experimented and you won't need to test as much as I did. I recommend that you do sufficient testing at the start to discover your peak time and then concentrate on testing at that time after each meal or snack. As you gain knowledge and your blood glucose levels improve you can gradually reduce the intensity of testing.

I consider the invention and development of the blood glucose test meter to be one of the true miracles of modern science for diabetes self-management; a wonderful benefit for all diabetics. But, sadly, after over three decades of continual meter development and improvement, the medical establishment does not understand how empowering home testing can be for their diabetic patients nor do doctors or educators teach patients this method.

That failure to educate is not really surprising when they have no idea of the possible benefits. Unfortunately there has never been a scientific study looking at this form of home testing. It is a method which has simply not occurred to the medical establishment.

As a consequence there are far too many doctors who see no value in home blood glucose testing and some doctors actively resist prescribing test strips to type 2 diabetics.

Reviewing for Good Nutrition

As you gradually improve your blood glucose levels you should also regularly review the resulting way of eating to ensure good nutrition. That includes checking for adequate minerals, vitamins, and fibre intake. If something is missing look for ways to include it in your menu without increasing blood glucose levels.

I know that I have a fairly well-balanced menu from past checks so I don't get obsessive about it. About every six months I use a diet analyser to do a detailed check on my daily menu. I have used several free analysers for that over the years. At the moment I use CRON-o-meter from http://spaz.ca/cronometer/. If that does not suit you there are many others on the web. I also have regular blood tests; those can also show if I am deficient in various vitamins and minerals. If analysis or blood tests show that I am missing something I then use the United States Department of Agriculture (USDA) nutrients guide: www.ars.usda.gov/Services/docs.htm?docid=8964.
That helps me find appropriate foods which provide those missing nutrients without increasing blood glucose levels.

In general terms I found that eating a variety of proteins such as meat, fish and eggs in normal, as against huge, serve sizes and replacing most of my starchy carbs, such as breads, potatoes, corn, pasta, rice and similar with a wide range of colourful vegetables, such as cabbage, spinach, celery, onions, peppers, lettuces, cauliflower, egg-plant, chard, broccoli, tomatoes and similar meant that there were very few nutrients I missed. In fact, the increased variety of foods, especially vegetables, in my diet improved my nutrient intake in many areas.

If, and only if, I cannot obtain a nutrient by adding a food to the menu I will add a supplement.

Adjust safely if you use medications

My signature on the web is "Everything in Moderation - Except Laughter". Do a search on that term and you will find me. That applies to everything I write.

Moderation is especially important if you use insulin or an insulin-stimulating medication and you start adjusting your carbohydrate portions. The insulin-stimulating medications include the sulfonylureas (such as Glimepiride, Glyburide and Glipizide) and the Meglitinides (such as Starlix and Prandin). There may be others on the market by the time you read this; if in doubt about your own medication ask your doctor or pharmacist. Metformin is not an insulin stimulator. If you use insulin or insulin-stimulating medications sudden changes from too many carbohydrates to too few can lead to changing your blood glucose levels from too high to too low. That is very unwise and can be dangerous.

If you are taking insulin or insulin-stimulating medications proceed cautiously after discussing this method with your doctor. Test after eating and if the result is high review the meal. Make a small change to the menu at the next meal of the same type. Repeat the process at that meal and continue with small changes, without risking hypos, until you see good numbers. Remember, you have time to make this work. There is no need to rush.

If you reach a stage where you feel your insulin or medication needs to be adjusted because your blood glucose levels are improving, discuss that with your doctor.

Testing Etiquette

After newly diagnosed diabetics have started using their meters to test after meals the next question is often "how can I test in public without embarrassing myself or upsetting others?"

I learned fairly early that my health was far more important than the sensibilities of spectators. That does not mean I make a spectacle of testing, or that I get aggressively "in-your-face" about it. I use a little tact and discretion, but I normally test anytime and anywhere I need to. I treat it as no different to blowing my nose or clearing my throat.

When I first applied the test, review, adjust technique

I tested publicly quite often. I found my peak timing by testing many times daily; I would set my watch count-down timer to alert me at that peak timing at the end of a meal or snack and when it went off I tested, usually regardless of where I was or who I was with. Of course I do not test as much these days because I can predict most results, but I still use that timer when I need to and I still test whenever it goes off.

No-one seeing me test has ever screamed or fainted or become upset in any way. In fact I occasionally met other diabetics when I tested and had some interesting chats; my blood glucose meter became a conversation piece.

If your friends have a problem with it, try to educate them. If that doesn't help, change your friends. Do you really want friends like them? If your relatives have a problem with it you can be a little blunter and drop some unsubtle hints about the genetic component of type 2. A few times relatives have commented and I offered to test them too; using a fresh lancet of course. For some of them that resulted in a need to see their doctor to confirm their own diagnosis. If it is your workplace then, of course, do not jeopardise employment. You will need to use your own judgement of the effect on employers and peers in that case. Sadly, ignorance will always exist in the real world and you must cater to it occasionally.

The only place I will NEVER test is in a place full of

possible infection: a public restroom or toilet, or a doctor's waiting room or similar high risk areas.

There are certain exceptions where a tactful delay is appropriate; but not a lot. It is your life. Literally. Test when and where you need to.

Testing on a Budget

I am very lucky to be in a country where diabetics in the past have successfully lobbied for specific support within the government health system to assist good diabetes control. I am eternally grateful to the pioneers who created Australian Medicare and the NDSS: the National Diabetes Services Scheme. If you are an Aussie you can find out more about the system if you go to their web-page at **www.ndss.com.au/**

However, I am daily reminded that diabetics overseas are not so fortunate. Consequently, some have difficulty following the full testing regimen I recommend because of the high cost of test strips.

If that applies to you, I suggest a basic "one strip a day" method. This works more slowly but it can still work. When I say "one strip a day" I am not counting the fasting blood glucose test or other tests the doctor wants. Discuss those with the doctor if you want to cut back there. In hard economic circumstances I cannot see that testing fasting blood glucose less often is going to be a major problem for the doctor, but check to be sure. Let's face it, the average type 2 is testing fasting blood glucose maybe once a week, doing absolutely nothing with the result, and wondering why their A1c goes up every 3 to 6 months.

This other daily test strip is purely to let YOU know what is really happening in your blood after you eat.

Before you commence it will take a few extra blood glucose tests over two or three days to discover when your peak occurs. Once you know that for each meal, you can focus on that timing. Some reckon you also need to test before meals to see what the rise was. In these circumstances I would see the pre-meal test as a waste of a test strip. Just concentrate on the absolute peak level. If you do not have enough strips to find your peak, then use one hour after you finish your meal as the test timing.

Target one meal per week. Most of us have problems with breakfast, so I recommend starting there.

Test at the peak spike time after breakfast each morning and use the test result to review the meal. Change your breakfast the next day to try to get a better result. Keep repeating that process for one week until you have modified your breakfast to the point where the after-meal blood glucose spikes are acceptable to you. I suggest you use the blood glucose guidelines listed in Appendix C as a guide. Concentrate on that meal for the first week; by that time you should have something workable.

I have given some alternative breakfast ideas in Chapter 10. Think outside the square and find what works for you. There is no law that decrees cereal, juice, milk or toast before noon; or at any time, for that matter.

Then concentrate on lunch for week two, dinner for week three and so on. Repeat that process over the next three weeks or check on snacks for a week or two. Then start again with breakfast. Over time you will find a range of foods that are OK - and a range of foods that are not - and slowly build a safe menu base.

All type 2 diabetics who start testing after meals discover fairly quickly that eating carbohydrates leads to a rise in blood glucose levels. That seems logical, and it is. So managing those carbohydrates and the resulting spikes becomes a cornerstone of their home treatment.

But pretty soon we also discover that logic has limitations. Some of us go to bed at night with good numbers and wake with high numbers. But we did not eat in our sleep. Or we make the mistake of thinking "food = spike, fasting = no spike" and find that after eating nothing for six hours we might be normal or even high when we expected to be low.

It does not seem to make sense, does it? So we start asking ourselves or our advisors "I ate nothing! Why are my blood glucose levels high?"

I do not pretend to be a medical expert or a bio-chemist, but I am pretty good at looking things up and testing the information I read against my own results. My body, my science experiment.

I checked this out a long time back when I first came across the term "liver dump", which is used by type 2 diabetics on the internet to describe the release of excessive energy from the liver to become blood glucose at times when we do not really need it or want it. Here is my version, based on distilling the information from several sources into something I can understand and relating that to the effects I have experienced myself.

Liver Dumps

We need glucose for energy. When we eat a meal it is usually a mix of carbohydrates, protein and fats. Carbohydrates are an easily converted source of energy which quickly appears as glucose in our blood as we digest our food. We also, more slowly, obtain glucose from protein or even fats using a process called gluconeogenesis, and also from the stored energy in our liver and other organs.

When we create more glucose than our immediate needs some is stored. Some is stored as fat, especially if we have excess insulin floating around, and some is converted to glycogen. Glycogen is stored mainly in the liver and the muscles. The muscles are selfish because the glycogen stored in the muscles can usually only be used for the muscles, but the glycogen stored in the liver is our supply for any glucose needed by the rest of the body. When a healthy body needs it the right amount is automatically released to the right places. As a result there is always a steady flow of energy to meet a person's needs, regulated to demand, regardless of when or what they eat.

Think of it as the body's version of a fuel tank.

At least, that is how it works in non-diabetics. Unfortunately, for type 2 diabetics, the system can be flawed.

Dawn Phenomenon

For example, one possible cause of the common problem called "Dawn Phenomenon", which occurs when we see high fasting blood glucose levels when we wake despite good numbers when we went to bed, is thought to be the body sensing our need for energy when we are about to wake, leading to excessive glycogen release until we eat and send the signal to stop the release. That is why a breakfast soon after we wake is an essential meal for many of us. Similarly, fasting for too long, strenuous exercise or heavy physical activity can lead to a liver dump if the body senses the reduction in blood glucose levels and over-compensates with excessive glycogen release.

Can we avoid liver dumps?

Preventing liver dumps is complex and I know no general solution. We all have to experiment to find our own individual solution.

For dawn phenomenon the most common treatment is to eat a late night snack. The reports of successful snacks vary widely so it is best to perform your own experiments until you find the one that works for you. I have seen everything from a glass of red wine, to a few olives, to some cheese, to a sandwich reported as successful. I eat a small serve of my Muesli, Nuts and Psyllium mix (see the Recipes Section) three or four nights a week. It works for me. Some people never have the problem, and a minority never find a food solution. Some of those have reported that a basal insulin was their solution.

The solution is easy for those who experience liver dumps after fasting. Do not fast for long periods. Eat something every few hours, even if it is only a small snack.

For those who get them during or after exercise, spreading small snacks across the period of exercise, including a snack before starting, can help.

It is not possible to be more specific with answers on dawn phenomenon or liver dumps. Once again it is your body, your science experiment.

Further reading

A good explanation of the "Dawn Phenomenon" and much more can be found in the misc.health.diabetes FAQ at www.faqs.org/faqs/diabetes/faq/

Load the page and scroll down to "Why is my morning bg high? What are dawn phenomenon, rebound, and Somogyi effect?"

WEIGHT LOSS

Chapter 8. Weight Loss Cooking and Eating Plan

Not all type 2 diabetics need to lose weight. If you are trim, taut and terrific, skip this chapter.

This is not so much a diet as a general guide to cooking and eating to help initially with weight loss; eventually leading to a sustainable longer-term way of eating. There are no absolutes; modify it to suit your own food likes and dislikes.

If you find any value in my experience, that is great. What follows was my own method of dealing with my own situation. I have passed it on to many people since I first wrote it. Many of those people used it to succeed with their own weight loss goals, but each changed it slightly to suit their own needs. I invite you to do the same.

It is also a work in progress because what I needed was to develop a "way of eating" that I could comfortably follow for the rest of my life; not just a short-term weight loss diet.

That is a point worth repeating. Short-term diets do not work. Science has repeatedly proved that. You may have discovered that yourself. You put in the effort, you try hard and you succeed in losing weight. And then, inexorably, it creeps back over the next few months or years. Why? Because you did not choose a way of life, you chose a short-term fix.

Instead, I chose to change some basic rules on the way I ate and lived; the most important one was that I never eat thoughtlessly now.

Use this in three stages.

Stage one is to apply the suggestions to your own favourite menus. Do not make drastic changes in types of food initially, just in portion sizes.

Stage two is to apply the suggestions in Chapter 6, Testing, Testing, to test those menu changes and their effects on your blood glucose levels. Remember that you are not just trying to lose weight; you are also trying to improve blood glucose levels. You have the opportunity to apply that immediately; I did not discover those techniques until months after I started my weight loss phase.

Stage Three is to gradually, over time, add new foods and variety to your menu and adjust portion sizes to achieve satiety or fullness without weight gain or blood glucose spikes.

When your desired weight loss is achieved some of the portion sizes may possibly be increased, but the general philosophy remains the same.

Background

The plan was developed over a few months after I was diagnosed with diabetes and leukaemia in early

2002. It is based on a distillation of research on the internet, advice from doctors, discussions with several dieticians and general reading on the subject over past years of yo-yo dieting. I had lost weight several times before, but it never stayed off.

I am 183cm (6') tall. In April 2002, at the time I was advised I had type 2 diabetes, I weighed 117 Kg or 257 lbs. By Christmas 2002 I weighed 94 Kg or 207 lbs, a loss of 23 Kg or 50 lbs. Equally important, I was reasonably fit, I did not feel hungry and I did not put it all back on over the Australian Christmas and New Year feasting period.

I wrote the first version of this in early 2003, when some friends on the CLL list asked for a copy of my "diet". I had to write it down for them because until that time it was just in my head. Since then I have travelled a lot, eaten out a lot, and learned a lot. And I have still kept the weight off. I have up-dated it since that first version to be more specific to type 2 diabetics, based on knowledge gained since the original version.

Long after I had successfully applied this I learned much more about fats, carbohydrates and protein and of the eternal diet wars between the low fat camp and the low carbohydrate camp. I am in the "whatever works for you" camp. Effectively I started with less of everything, except for vegetables, compared to the way I used to eat.

This is only the starting point. As time goes on and weight comes off the constraints on fat can be eased but your meter will probably show you that the constraints on carbohydrates tend to remain.

I will stay out of the diet wars and simply say that this worked for me at that time and has worked for many others since.

WEIGHT LOSS PLAN

Reduce Meat Portion Sizes

Start by halving your meat portions and then adjust as required.

Almost all of us eat meat and protein serves that are far too big. In our affluent society we have become accustomed to portion sizes at each meal that would feed a family for a week in the third world. Over time I settled on some standard sizes for myself. My chicken portion is equivalent to a thigh or half a breast; my steak would be less than the size of a deck of cards; two lamb chops is a full serve and my pork chop is cut in half and shared with my wife.

Cut Back on Red Meat Portions

Replace many of your red meat portions with fish. I have no portion size limit for fish. I do not have anything against red meat, it is a great source of many good nutrients such as iron and the B vitamins and I still eat it at over half of my meals, but fish has many other benefits as well as usually being leaner. The oils in fish are mainly good oils, high in omega 3.

Increase Omega 3 Fish Meals

Add salmon, sardines, tuna, mackerel and similar oily fish to the menu, preferably fresh rather than canned. However, if canned is all you can economically get, then that will do provided that there are no health problems with the canned fish available in your region.

In addition to oily fish, include other forms of fish and seafood in your menu. Most of us eat breakfast, lunch and dinner every day, which means we eat at least 21 main meals per week. Try to include fish in at least seven of those meals.

Increase Vegetable serves

This is where you can eat to your heart's content. Literally. Start with your favourites but try to expand the variety and range of your vegetable serves. Cabbage, celery, broccoli, spinach, silver-beet (chard) and similar vegetables are your friends.

Minimise Milk

Minimise all types of milk, regardless of fat content. My only exception was yoghurt. Skim milk may actually cause bigger blood glucose spikes because of the slightly higher carbohydrate content and lack of fat.

For cheese, I eat full-fat cheese but less of it. I cannot stand most of the "plastic" manufactured low fat cheeses. There are some cheeses with lower fat content that I use in dips such as cottage, ricotta or low fat Philadelphia Cheese where I can add flavours; my "Cheesy Guacamole" is an example in the Recipes section. Take calcium supplements if necessary and appropriate to replace the loss of dairy calcium. Be aware that there can be lots of calcium in green vegetables so add more of those first. I also added Greek yoghurt, which helped add calcium and had other benefits.

Later, when I had achieved my weight loss, I added more cheeses back into my menu. I like aged cheddars, brie, camembert, blue vein and parmesan, among others. But I was strict about portion sizes while losing the weight.

Good Snacks

Avoid starchy and sugary snacks or processed food bars. See Chapter 12, Snacks, for some ideas on snacks that will fill the "I've gotta eat something" gap without leading to increases in either the waist-line or blood glucose levels.

Variety

Vary your meals and menus as much as possible to prevent boredom. Experiment by creating tasty dips for snacks, adding unusual spices to casseroles or marinades and trying new or different recipes. But always have a stand-by in the freezer to allow for the occasional inedible disaster.

Guilt and Failure

Allow yourself a "guilt-free" day or meal occasionally. Pizza, fish and chips (deep-fried battered fish with french fries for those people who drive on the wrong side of the road), chocolates etc. However, still apply common sense and try to keep the portion size reasonable or cook it at home where you can control the fat and carbohydrate content. Yes, I know it is impossible to eat one chocolate out of a full box. But try. If you allow this luxury it makes it easier to return to the plan, rather than to think "well I have blown it now, so what the heck!"

Saturated Fat Elimination/Reduction

My use of fats and oils has changed and increased after I achieved my weight loss and I changed to a long-term way of eating. Now that I have lost the weight I no longer worry as much about fats. However, this section is based honestly on the techniques I used back then to lose the weight. I realise that some people will always worry about fats no matter what, so I have left these tips in.

Trim all fresh meats carefully to discard as much fat as possible. Grill (broil for Americans) meats when possible so that fats drain during cooking. Do not use processed meat; for example avoid all sausages, salami, bologna, processed chicken rolls and similar until you achieve your target weight.

Do not eat take-away chips or fries or similar deep-fried fast foods. If you're caught with a group at a take-away have salad (watch the dressing), skin-free chicken or just a very small serve. More take-away restaurants are offering salads now. Another alternative for take-away restaurants is to substitute deli sandwiches. However, be careful with the bread portion; I often discard all the bread or at least the top piece.

Good Oils

We need some oils for good health. The problem is that I used to eat far too much of everything, including the good oils. I reduced those as well but I continue to use oils such as extra virgin olive oil, canola, peanut oil and similar for cooking. I eat avocado without restraint and nuts in moderation.

Fat Reduction in Cooking

Use cooking sprays instead of butter or spoonfuls of oil for cooking. Use a thin smear of whole-egg mayo or a spread you like instead of margarine or butter on sandwiches or rolls and do not have the top half of the bun or the top slice of bread. Experiment. Cook casseroles in advance and cool in the refrigerator. The saturated fat will rise to the top and solidify and can be removed before re-heating or thickening. As an alternative, strain the liquid and cool it separately before re-combining. Reduced fat gravies can be made from pan juices by pouring them off into a jug, letting them settle until the fat rises to the top and then skimming. Add some ice cubes to speed up the process if the diners are waiting. The juices will still contain fat, but not as much.

Use a non-stick pan or griddle; I use a seasoned cast-iron skillet. Most meats will not need additional oil to cook, or will only need a light spray from cooking oil. If you must deep-fry (a rare luxury – see "guilt-free" days) use a vegetable oil, preferably peanut or another high smoke point oil and wait until the oil is at the correct temperature before adding the food. Do not over-crowd the pan as this reduces the temperature and causes the food to absorb more oil. Drain the fried food well on kitchen paper before serving. When I say it is a luxury, I fried fish once a fortnight but I oven fried the chips.

Oven fry french fries. Cut them large, not like thin fast-food fries, parboil them in boiling water until not quite cooked but still firm, spray an oven tray with cooking oil then place the "fries" on the tray and spray again lightly. Cook in the oven at about 200C (390F) until done. Use your meter to see what portion size you can handle. Mine is three chips.

Sugars and Sweeteners

I won't buy into the arguments about sweeteners in this book, although I have written about them on my blog. People say some may give you cancer. Do you think that worries a Diabetic Leukemic? Find the sweetener and lo-cal drink that you like, or that you dislike least, and consider all foods flavoured with sugar as poison until you have tested those foods with your meter. If you must eat them, make it a special and rare treat.

Carbohydrates

You may think you need carbohydrates for energy, fibre and brain food but steer clear of the white starches. I eat a moderate intake of grains, cereals and legumes to keep me regular and provide variety in my diet but I found my limits for those foods by using my meter. Until you know those limits, treat all carbohydrates with caution.

Add other sources of fibre, particularly leafy or green vegetables. I also add psyllium husk to my menu for extra fibre without extra calories or blood glucose spikes.

Drinks

I drink water, diet soft drinks, red wine, tea and coffee. Do not drink anything with a high sugar content, including milk (lactose). Check soy milk for fat and sugar content. Be very wary of vegetable juices and cut all fruit juices; basically they are concentrated fruit without the fibre and will send your blood glucose levels sky-high. Coffee is acceptable in moderation but be careful of adding milk or, worse, artificial creamers.

Alcohol

Alcohol is a very personal issue, so that is one to be discussed directly with your doctor. Personally, I drink two or three glasses of good red wine a day as I discuss in Chapter 16. One of the pleasant things I discovered by blood glucose testing is that a good red wine helps reduce my numbers. Unfortunately, you can have too much of a good thing. I have the occasional scotch or rum and diet mixer. This is probably more than the doctor would recommend but, as I have learnt, life is too short to give up all the good things. Remember – everything in moderation.

Nutrition Labels

Learn to read nutrition labels on the packet. Until you start to read them you do not realise how much variation there is in the fat, carbohydrate and sugar content of the products you buy. Modify your purchasing habits as a result. If a product is advertised as low fat or low-cal but there is no nutrition detail it is probably misleading advertising.

Be very wary of "lite" or "97% fat-free" and similar claims; they often compensate for the reduced fat by increasing the level of sugar or HFCS (a sweetener used in America made from corn) and can contain more calories than the standard product. Also remember that "sugar-free" is not usually carb-free or even carb-reduced.

Discipline

Set a healthy target in consultation with your medical advisors then set smaller targets on the way to your goal. Celebrate in some way each time you reach the target. I used 2kg as my small goal and 10kg as a major celebration goal. Broad equivalent goals for US readers would be 5lbs and 20lbs.

Involve those you care about so that they can encourage you. It won't work if you quit, and you will quit if you do not get results. Weigh yourself regularly and record the results. Do not get dejected if your waistline or weight does not go down every day. The body seems to take time to adjust to the changes. In my case I lost 3 Kg (6 ½ lbs) in the first week, but this stabilised to an average of about a kilo per week and later to half a kilo. There were some weeks or months when I seemed to hover or even go up, but then I would lose a lot in the next week.

FOOD, GLORIOUS FOOD

Over the years I have spent reading and writing on various diabetes forums I have noticed that people seem to fall into one of three broad categories when it comes to working in the kitchen. There are those who cook for themselves and enjoy doing it; those who cannot cook and who survive on someone else's cooking at home or in a restaurant, or who eat pre-packaged or ready-made foods; and those who can cook but do not enjoy it and only do it when they have no alternative.

My research after diagnosis led me to two unsurprising revelations for an obese Type 2 diabetic. I needed to lose a lot of weight and I needed to control my blood glucose. Of course, there are other factors, but those two were paramount.

I believe it was much easier for me to achieve reasonable weight and blood glucose control moderately swiftly because I am a person who enjoys cooking. That allows me to be the one who controls what goes into the recipe by type and quantity, to control the size of portions and to experiment by testing the results.

I can only imagine the stress it places on a relationship when the diabetic is trying to tactfully tell the cook that the new dish or dessert that they made with love is either too many carbohydrates or so full of artificial sweeteners it tastes horrible and that the real problem is the flour, not the sugar, anyway. Or that they now need five meals or snacks a day including a cooked breakfast; and so on. A major chronic condition places enough stress on relationships without that.

I have also noticed a continual search by those who do not cook for "safe" pre-prepared foods in the supermarket, "low carbohydrate" this and "sugar free" that, or "safe" fast foods and restaurant foods.

Fast foods or pre-prepared foods are convenient and I know that some people are forced to eat out by work or local social requirements. However, there is no doubt in my mind that the easiest way to control your own diet is to be the person who creates the menu and cooks the dishes on it.

Basic home cooking is not that difficult. One reason I have included some example recipes is to show that. All of my recipes are simple and basic with reasonably short lists of the sort of ingredients found in most homes.

Practice, experiment, and do not get upset if you have an inedible failure. That is why you cooked extra the time before so there was something in the freezer for a quick zap in the microwave.

Chapter 10. Breakfasts

Breakfast is a difficult meal which deserves a chapter of its own.

There are few more serious errors in the present advice given by nutritionists and dieticians to new type 2 diabetics than to eat the traditional "heart-healthy" breakfast of cereal, milk, toast or bagel, washed down by a fruit juice or a glass of milk. In effect, sugared starch, with a side of starch, washed down by sugar.

I am one of the many type 2 diabetics who found that breakfast was the hardest meal of the day to get right.

There are also few meals more difficult for people to change. Old habits based on cereal, milk, juice and oatmeal learned in our childhood around our mother's table can be extremely difficult to break. Despite popular opinion to the contrary, those rules for breakfast ingredients are not actually mandatory.

Additionally, a significant number of people do not eat breakfast at all. That is not a good idea for a type 2 diabetic; I give the reasons for that in Chapter 7, Dawn Phenomenon and Liver Dumps.

After a lot of personal experimentation I came up with some ideas for myself as alternatives to the traditional overload of carbohydrates at breakfast. Use them as a base for your own ideas, adjusting for your own likes and dislikes. Or think up some of your own using your favourite low-carbohydrate foods.

Eggs

The humble egg can be cooked in so many ways: poached, fried, normal omelette, fluffy omelette (separate the yolks, whip the white with a spoonful of water, fold back with filling and yolks), scrambled with a little milk, frittata (a heavier omelette with filling), quiche and baked. Use vegetable fillings or cheese and add fresh herbs if you can or dried herbs if you can't.

When breakfast is discussed on diabetes forums, especially forums in the USA, many people mention using egg whites, "egg-beaters" or other yolk-less forms of eggs. When I query them on their reasons, their fear is almost always that the cholesterol in eggs would raise their serum cholesterol levels.

It appears that they may be partially correct if you eat a low fat diet, but if you eat eggs as part of a reduced carbohydrate diet the cholesterol that is raised is the good cholesterol, HDL.

That is the conclusion of a study titled "Dietary Cholesterol from Eggs Increases Plasma HDL Cholesterol in Overweight Men Consuming a Carbohydrate-Restricted Diet" in J. Nutr. 138:272-276,

February 2008.

I do not want to infringe copyright so I invite you to read it yourself. It is online at this url: http://jn.nutrition.org/cgi/content/abstract/138/2/272 I received permission from the authors to include some selected snippets; I liked the wording of the approval message: "feel free to quote those paragraphs. You got the idea correctly".

"Carbohydrate-restricted diets significantly decrease body weight and independently improve plasma triglycerides and HDL cholesterol.
And:
These results suggest that including eggs in a Carbohydrate-restricted diet results in increased HDL-C while decreasing the risk factors associated with Metabolic Syndrome."

Have an omelette for breakfast tomorrow and also notice the improvement in your peak after-breakfast blood glucose tests.

Eggs are also a great breakfast for those in a hurry in the morning. Here are a couple of quick and easy examples.

Instant Scrambled Eggs

In a hurry? Or is your only cooking tool available at breakfast time a microwave? This is for you.

Break an egg or two into a mug or cup, add a splash of milk, season to taste, beat lightly with a fork and microwave it for 60 seconds on high. Check, stir, and repeat in 15 second bursts if necessary. The time needed varies because microwave powers vary. After the first time you will know how long to set it for. Save on washing up time by eating direct from the mug with the fork you used to stir it.

If you want to get fancy, a little chopped parsley or your own favourite herb added before cooking is good.

Omelette

Put your skillet on moderate heat. Break two or three eggs into a bowl, add a splash (a tablespoonful or less) of water, season to taste, whisk briefly with a fork, add a little oil or butter or both to the skillet and pour in the egg mix. Use the same fork to gently move the liquid from the edges to the centre and vice-versa and as soon as it is not quite set fold it over and serve. The whole process should take less than five minutes from opening the pantry door to sitting down to eat.

Meats

Consider bacon, ham, small steaks, hamburger patties, chicken, prosciutto and similar meats. They can be fried, grilled or broiled. They can also be chopped, cooked and added to omelettes or frittata or scrambled eggs. For bacon or other fatty meats, drain on absorbent paper before serving if you wish to reduce the fat.

Fish

Try fish smoked, canned or fresh. It can be poached, fried, cooked in a mornay (go easy on the thickener), mixed in a stir-fry or any other way you like it. The same logic applies to seafood.

Mushrooms

Small mushrooms can be sliced and cooked with onions, herbs, garlic and a little oil and a smidgin of flour or guar gum for a gravy. Large ones can be filled with bolognaise or napoli sauce (or whatever you like), topped with grated cheese and baked in the oven. Sliced fried mushrooms are also another good omelette filling.

Casseroles and stews

Try beef, lamb, chicken, mince (ground beef), or whatever is your favourite. Check the carbohydrates in the recipe to check suitability. If you get a blood glucose spike the culprits will usually be thickeners or root vegetables.

The casserole or stew can be pre-prepared and divided, after cooking and cooling, into individual breakfast sized serves. Put them in small plastic containers in the freezer and when you need a quick and easy breakfast zap one in the microwave. My favourites are Beef Burgundy or Breakfast Stew, but you should make your own favourites.

Leftovers

I often have an egg with a re-heated lamb chop, or slices of roast meat or similar left-overs for a quick breakfast.

Use your imagination when looking for better breakfasts. Always do an after-meal blood glucose test the first time you try a new breakfast to be sure you have chosen the right portion size.

Chapter 11. Grazing

Another lady who added a lot to my diabetes knowledge was "Ozgirl". I met her in cyberspace some years ago on the alt.support.diabetes newsgroup. It was Ozgirl who introduced me to "grazing" as a blood glucose management tool. She developed her own method to combat her reactive hypoglycemia and I found that the method was very effective for me to minimise after-meal blood glucose spikes. I have since met her in real life, she is an Aussie Super-mum who practises what she preaches, looking after both her diabetes and her large family incredibly well.

If eating traditional sized meals at traditional times is not working for you, grazing may be an option for you to consider.

As a diabetic one of my goals is to try to keep my blood glucose levels stable and as close to normal as I can. I found that eating the traditional "three square meals" daily caused problems and it became much easier when I broke those meals up into a series of smaller meals and snacks. Dinner is still my biggest meal, but the others are all small. A side benefit is that I rarely feel hungry.

My day goes something like this:

Morning: breakfast, as soon as possible after waking

Mid-morning: a small snack.

Around noon: a small lunch

Mid-afternoon: a small snack.

Evening: dinner

An hour or two after dinner: a small snack. This is usually my after-dinner dessert.

Bedtime: A small supper.

Effectively I rarely go more than three hours without eating something, but the portion I eat is very small. When I say a small snack, I mean the equivalent of half an apple or a cracker with cheese or a half-cup of yoghurt with berries. Those are typical portion sizes that my meter showed did not cause blood glucose spikes between meals. Breakfast is equivalent to an egg or two and a thick slice of ham or a rasher of bacon; lunch an open sandwich, or a soup, or a stir-fry or similar. Snacks are small, as described in the next chapter.

The total calories in the day are the same but they are spread across the time more evenly.

Chapter 12. Snacks

It can be difficult to find snacks that will meet the need for some quick nourishment without raising blood glucose levels or adding to the waistline. Here are a few ideas based on my own menu and test results. Experiment; base your choices on the foods you like and develop your own choices to fill those "gotta have something" moments or to help you graze.

Nuts

Nuts are an excellent snack if eaten as an occasional handful. My preferred mix is unsalted roasted cashews, brazils, hazelnuts, almonds and walnuts or pecans. Peanuts are not nuts, they are legumes. I avoid salted nuts or salted peanuts because salt can create thirst and also leads to a tendency to empty the whole bowl. The old adage that it is impossible to eat just one salted nut from a full bowl is too true.

Olives

Eat them in any form you like. I stopped buying pitted olives because I ate too many at a time. I found that eating whole marinated olives slowed down my snacking because it takes a little longer when you have to munch around the seed. I buy them cheaply in large bottles and add chopped hot chilli, onion and herbs to the bottle to flavour them.

Dips

Pre-made supermarket dips can be good, but check labels for carbohydrate content. It is easy to make your own. Experiment with your favourite vegetables, chopped and mixed with creamy cheeses, herbs and flavours such as ginger or garlic. See my cheesy guacamole dip recipe as an example to modify to your own taste. Also consider other dips such as hummus or guacamole. Low-carbohydrate crackers can be used as dippers, but it can be difficult to stop if it is a tasty dip and the carbohydrate load can sneak up on you. It is better to use strips of crisp vegetables such as carrot or celery for dipping.

Half portions of fruit

A half portion of an apple, orange, pear or similar can fill that gap without leading to a **blood glucose** spike. The leftovers become another snack later in the day. A full piece of a smaller fruit such as a peach or nectarine can also be a quick snack. Use your meter to find the right snack portion sizes for the fruits you like.

Left-over salad from an earlier meal

Deliberately leave a little over in the salad bowl after a meal to be a quick and easy between-meals snack, dressed with a little balsamic vinegar and extra-virgin olive oil or with whole-egg mayo.

Crackers

Crackers can be fine provided you are aware of their carbohydrate content. I use a version that is 6 gms carbohydrate per cracker. Use whatever cracker-topping you like as long it is a small portion and not too high in carbohydrates.

Avocado

Avocado is an excellent food, low in carbohydrates but full of good oils and healthy vitamins and minerals. For a quick snack I slice a small to medium avocado in half, twist so that I have a free portion and a seed portion, store the seed half in the fridge for later on, sprinkle a little salt and maybe a squirt of lime-juice on the other half and eat it direct from the shell with a teaspoon. If it is a big avocado I may get four serves out of one. Another option is to mash a half-avocado and some grated parmesan cheese with a fork, add salt and pepper and a splash of citrus to create instant guacamole. Spread it on a cracker or use it as a dip.

In this fast, convenience society of ours we eat out much more often than our parents did.

Since I was diagnosed with type 2 diabetes I have travelled the world and visited many countries. I have eaten almost every cuisine you can imagine including North, Central and South America, China, South-East Asia, India, Europe and the Middle East. Each trip was months long and every meal was eating out. Despite that, I did not put on weight and my blood glucose levels were good as I travelled. Here are some of the tips and tricks I developed to make sure I do not undo the good work I have done at home when I am eating out.

Be strong

We were brought up to clean our plate, not to waste food. But now, that "waste not, want not" attitude to the food on our plate can kill us. Be strong enough to leave food on your plate even though you paid good money for it.

Order wisely

Check the menu to see what side orders automatically accompany the main course. If items such as rice, fries, pasta or other starches are on the list ask the waiter to delete those or to substitute vegetables or salad. If you do not check in advance and the side orders appear on the table it is human nature to eat them, even if you intended not to. It is much easier to not let them appear in the first place.

When eating alone it can be useful to ignore the main course menu and choose only from the soup or appetiser menu. If one appetiser is not enough, have two or a soup and an appetiser. The appetisers often have a wider range of flavours and they are rarely overloaded with potato or rice or pasta. You need to be a bit more careful with some soups. Avoid thickened soups because many chefs use cornstarch or similar for the thickener.

In the USA, UK and Australia I very rarely order a main course when eating alone. In other countries the serve sizes tend to be smaller but I still often leave food on the plate.

No fries

Make it clear to the waiter that you absolutely do NOT want chips or fries even though they may be included with the meal. Often they will substitute vegetables or salad if you ask. If unwanted foods appear it can sometimes help if you transfer them to a side plate and then try to ignore them.

Fast food

Avoid fast-food franchises where possible. In some countries they can be useful for other things such as clean conveniences. In that case I order the least dangerous food item on their menu to "pay" for using the facilities; whether or not I eat it depends on the situation. I quite liked McAloo Tikki in India the one time I tried it at one of their Golden Arches restaurants. Later, I read the nutrition detail when I got home. I won't be trying it again.

When fast food is the only choice, be strong again. Order a salad if that is available, or eat the burger and toss the bun. Do not order up. Do not drink post-mix sodas; you have no control over which button the waiter presses or even which line is connected to the diet soda when they run out of diet syrup. If you cannot buy a bottle or can, then drink water or coffee or tea, with sweetener if necessary. Note that a teaspoon of sugar you add yourself is not likely to be a big problem, but the amount they add to a cup of iced tea or a regular soda is.

Avoid special orders

Never ask for diabetic or low carb meals. Both will only confuse your waiter and the former is likely to be the highest carbohydrate meal at your table. It is better to pick the best you can from the menu and do what you can to modify it easily, such as substituting salad or vegetables for fries or similar foods.

Test, test, test

If you eat at a restaurant you are likely to return to, be sure to test at your peak afterwards to see what happened. That may affect your decision on returning or your menu selection when you do. Test, do not guess. The results will sometimes surprise you. The quantity of sugar, HFCS or starches that may be added to some savoury recipes which are not obviously sweet is quite amazing.

Sharing

When I am travelling with my wife, eating out is much simpler. On two trips around the world together we left a reputation behind us as Aussie cheapskates because, wherever we went, we would order one main course and a spare plate for the two of us. It took some cheek, but we did not put the weight back on. We also saved some cash, but that was a bonus, not the intention. Where it was not practicable because of language difficulties or possible embarrassment of others we would order a main course and a side salad or starter – just to get the plate – then mix between the two. This allowed me to leave the high carbohydrate items for my non-diabetic wife. We often found that we still left food on the plate, even when we shared. The food is actually the smallest cost in running most restaurants; many chefs provide enormous serves to attract return customers.

Breakfasts

Hotel breakfasts can vary from wonderful buffet choices to disastrous "continental" breakfasts of a tired croissant and grey cold imitation coffee. They can also be incredibly expensive, with minimum prices in the restaurant or high extras and tips on room service. I refuse to pay through the nose for some watery scrambled eggs and a coffee. If the hotel choice is OK or I can cook my own, wonderful; if not I have a standard routine on arrival at a hotel.

I ask at reception where the nearest diners, cafés and restaurants are. If appropriate I ask for the hotel staff's recommendations. At an appropriate time after I check in, usually after dinner, I take a walk around the district. If I arrived by car I will have already been watching for restaurants and diners as I drove in. I use the walk for exercise and also to check out a likely place for breakfast. It is rare that there are no diners or similar within a reasonable walk. That walk can also double as my morning exercise.

Asian cuisine

If in Asia, or an Asian restaurant, leave almost all of the rice on the plate. Also limit breads like Naan or Roti. I can handle a roti or a half-Naan at dinner but only if I do not have rice. Be wary of some of the popular sweeter Indian dishes such as butter chicken, also known as chicken makhani, which can have a very high sugar content. Similarly be cautious about

Chinese sweet-and-sour or honey or plum sauce dishes and soups thickened with cornstarch. If in doubt eat a small serve the first time and test to see what your limits are next time you try that dish.

Whenever you eat out always remember that the portion sizes on your plate are chosen by the chef to entice you to return, not by your doctor to improve your health.

Money can be tight in these troubled and uncertain times. As well as medical costs, this response I received from a newly diagnosed type 2 when I suggested adding more vegetables and fish to a menu is typical of many: "But eating lower carbohydrate versions of food is EXPENSIVE. I know some people say that eating healthy is not any more expensive than eating cheap but they are full of it."

I suppose where you live has a lot to do with that. However, how you manage your time and resources can affect it too.

I found that I actually saved money when we started "eating healthy". But I had to work at it, because it takes a little planning and effort. To start with, I ate less than I did in the past; significantly less for some foods. That did not cover the higher costs of some new foods like asparagus, avocado and similar, but I certainly saved on breads, potatoes, corn, rice and similar starches. I also saved a lot on meat, by eating a lot less than I did in the past, and by not purchasing a lot of processed sauces and packet foods.

Money is not everything; there are other costs such as time. I accepted that part of the price for better health was a little more time spent in the kitchen. I also accepted some additional inconvenience.

Cooking more often at home also saves on the costs of eating out or fast-foods. It is always cheaper to cook at home even if you cook the same things as the fast-food places such as hamburgers or fried fish. But it does take more time and work.

There are also ways to use time more efficiently. As I was already spending more time in the kitchen I looked at ways of economising money and time. One major way to do that is to both buy and cook in bulk. An investment in a freezer and microwave will repay you many times over in being able to buy ingredients in season when prices are low and store them appropriately for later use.

I buy meats and fish in bulk. Our supermarkets and butchers often have "specials" if the customer buys at least two or three kilos. For example, I usually buy a "full rump" (flank steak), which is about five or six kilos (11-14lbs) as an uncut lump of meat from the butcher at a much cheaper price than the cut and trimmed beef. At home I slice the premium parts, trimmed of fat, into a large number of small 100gm (3 to 4oz) steaks. I trim the scrappier bits and cut them roughly into 2.5cm (1") cubes for stews. I then cling-wrap each individual steak and two-cup lots of stew chunks for freezing for future use. When I need a steak in the future it is there in the freezer ready for me. Sometimes I buy much cheaper cuts in bulk such as gravy beef or stewing steak just for casseroles.

Later I spend an afternoon cooking up stews,

casseroles and soups in bulk, freezing the results in single-serve containers. When it comes time to eat those I have got a meal via the microwave in minutes that is cheaper, faster, healthier and tastier than anything from a fast-food restaurant. I do the same thing for fish, chicken and pork, waiting until "specials" appear for bulk lots or a seasonal glut occurs.

Many vegetables and fruits can be bulk cooked and frozen too. I buy or grow in season vegetables like tomatoes, silver-beet (a type of swiss chard, a good spinach alternative), sweet corn (I blanch and freeze 1/3 cob portions), string beans and several others. I buy mango, which can be very cheap in season here, or berries, and freeze those for later addition to home-made yoghurt.

As well as eating less I waste less. The change in the level of waste in our rubbish bin was quite dramatic when we stopped buying processed packet foods and also started being stricter for portion sizes; allied to that we are much more aware of separating scraps for the compost bin to help grow some of our own vegetables. That is another way to save on food costs for those with the luxury of some backyard or even planter pot space to do so.

We, as a couple, took the time to compare grocery bills from before my diagnosis and a couple of years later. Despite inflation, we were paying slightly less for our weekly food while eating healthier and tastier.

In the end, everything has a price. The cost may be calculated in dollars, health, time, or some other currency. What it boils down to is whether the goals we set for ourselves are worth the price. Each of us has to make that decision, but it helps if you truly calculate the cost.

You will find that many people claim benefits from using cinnamon to reduce blood glucose peaks. Many of the stories about cinnamon can be traced back to a limited study in Pakistan a few years ago and some US follow-ups. I won't argue about their validity but I have seen no credible in-depth studies on the subject. However, it keeps recurring almost weekly on places like the ADA forum and similar diabetes forums.

The minimal, if any, effect that cinnamon had on me was trivial. Reducing my carbohydrate input by just a few grams had a much greater effect. I still use cinnamon as a spice frequently and infuse it in my morning coffee - but for taste, not blood glucose improvements. It did affect my after-breakfast blood glucose peak indirectly because I no longer add milk to my morning coffee as a consequence.

That does not mean that spices and herbs should not be used. In fact I recommend you include them regularly in your menu. I use many herbs and spices. Some for taste, some for medicinal purposes, some for both. Some have proven benefits, such as turmeric for some cancers, some are anecdotal. My attitude is that if it is not harmful I have nothing to lose and a possible gain by adding such things to my menu. However, I do not buy capsules or pills of cinnamon, or turmeric, or garlic or similar supplements. I eat them by including the herbs, spices and specific foods regularly in my normal way of eating. I sometimes include them by spicing up an existing recipe, such as a sprinkle of turmeric and black pepper (the two are complementary) in a morning omelette; sometimes by adding new spicy dishes to my menu, such as Asian stir-fries, and sometimes just to add a little variation to an old favourite dish.

I have tiny amounts of many things almost every day.

As I wrote this I reviewed the herbs and spices in my menu over the last few days; just normal days, nothing unusual. In that brief time I included turmeric, cinnamon, nutmeg, grated black pepper, cumin, paprika, thyme, mint, basil, rosemary, hot chilli, fresh garlic, grated ginger and the broad combination spices of garam masala and commercial curry powder. That is in addition to ensuring my menu also included items like avocado, nuts, psyllium husks, leafy greens, onions, capsicum (bell peppers) and several other good foods. Most of my herbs are grown fresh at home. When the crop is over-abundant I dry it, chop it and store it for future use out of season.

As to which of those, if any, is helping my diabetes or my CLL, who knows. I'll follow my doctors' advice and keep doing what I am doing. Even if they do not improve my health, they definitely help a slightly re-stricted menu taste delicious.

Chapter 16. Red, Red Wine

I am a believer in the value of a modest intake of alcohol in the form of red wine.

Some people cannot drink alcohol because they have addiction or other medical or ideological reasons for abstinence. For the rest of us the evidence is becoming fairly clear that a moderate regular intake of alcohol is beneficial, particularly for type 2 diabetics. The benefits appear to be enhanced if the alcohol of choice is red wine.

I usually drink dry red wine. I have found that many people do not understand the term "dry". It simply means "not sweet". Sweet wines such as lambrusco, dolcetto or most white wines and fortified or dessert wines such as ports, sherry, madeira and tokay are not suitable for me because the sugars in them raise my blood glucose. The only white wines I can drink are the very dry Sauvignons Blanc or Chablis styles.

In essence I drink dry red wine for the following reasons:

1. I like red wine. That is important. If you do not like wine, do not start. I shudder at the thought of having to "take it as a medicine".

2. Red wine appears to assist in my blood glucose

control when taken with meals.

3. Red wine appears to improve my cardiovascular health, based on my own lab reports since I added it to my menu after diagnosis.

4. Red wines include some specific benefits over other alcoholic drinks because of their unique resveratrols and flavonoids.

If you search the web you will find many studies which tend to support the possibility that I am not unique in seeing those benefits.

Any proposed changes in your alcohol consumption should first be discussed with your doctor. There may be other reasons for abstinence, apart from addiction, that your doctor is aware of. However, do not automatically accept warnings against alcohol on medication packets. Instead, discuss those with your doctor to see if it applies in your individual situation.

The various studies are not in agreement on "moderation". The definition appears to lie between one and three "standard" glasses daily for a male and half that for a female. Sorry, ladies, I know that is unfair but when our bodies were designed no-one told the designer that was discrimination.

USEFUL INFORMATION

Sometimes it may take a few days to get organised and arrange to get your new meter. Or you may already have a meter but you are still deciding whether to follow the testing suggestions in this book. That is OK, take your time. It is an important decision. Think about it for a while and discuss it with your medical advisors.

What follows are some suggestions to help you get started in the right direction. This is not intended as suggestions for a permanent menu. It is intended as a temporary measure until systematic blood glucose testing can be started. It will also be useful as a basic initial shopping guide.

These broad guidelines should help minimise after-meal blood glucose spikes without jeopardising overall nutrition.

If you are using insulin or an insulin-stimulating medication such as a sulfonylurea you should discuss these suggestions with your doctor. But if you are using insulin or those medications you should also have a meter and have received training on the relationship between insulin or medications and carbohydrates. If that is not the case, ask your diabetes educator why not.

Minimise:

Anything made in a bakery.

Pasta.

Rice.

All wheat products.

All corn products.

All cereals and other processed grains.

Starches - especially root vegetables.

All sugared drinks - sodas, sport drinks, milk.

All juices, both fruit and vegetable.

All fast foods.

All processed or packet foods.

At this stage, when choosing foods ignore food colour, fibre content or advertising hype about wholegrain, low-GI or low sugar foods. You can use your meter to check the validity of those claims later.

Be Wary of:

Fruits, which can be good in small portions but may cause quite high blood glucose levels if consumed in large portions. My own limit is equivalent to a half-apple or a half orange as a between-meals snack.

Maximise:

All vegetables, apart from root vegetables.

Eat in moderate portions:

Fish.
Meats.
Eggs.
Beans.
Nuts.
Avocado.

Those lists are not exhaustive but I think you will see
the trends.

One of the common objections to self-testing blood glucose more frequently is a fear of pain from testing. If you are suffering pain when you test then you are doing it incorrectly.

I learned this the hard way in my first year after diagnosis. I hope it helps you.

If possible, wash your hands in warm water first and shake them to get the circulation going. If that is not possible I know where my fingers have been so I use what I call the "KFC" method: finger-lickin'-good.

Check your lancet-holder; it should be adjustable. Mine is a Multi-clix, made by Roche and is usually painless. My earlier lancet was the Soft-clix, also by Roche. That brand has an excellent reputation among the diabetics I know, but any good lancet device should do the job. I get an occasional tiny sting and it lets me know if it is getting blunt sometimes but I tested over 5,000 times in the first four years after diagnosis, before I stopped counting, without any trauma. That is from a guy who was, and is, needle-phobic.

Start with the second lowest setting of 1 or 1.5. Press the business end of the lancet device reasonably firmly against your skin on the side of a finger near the tip. Do not flinch when you release the button.

The button releases a spring-loaded tiny needle which makes a tiny hole in your skin and instantly retracts. Using the side of your finger-tip has two advantages: there are less nerve-ends than on the pads and it doubles the number of test-points so you can rotate through them.

Do not squeeze too hard; instead massage gently from the base to the tip of the finger until a drop of blood forms sufficient to apply to the test strip. Squeezing too hard may add interstitial fluid to the blood droplet and affect the result. If this setting does not provide an adequate sample move the lancet setting up one notch for the next one. If you got a large sample and it hurt a little, go to the next lower setting.

And that is all there is to it. Sometimes it helps to shake your hands a little more, or warm them up if it is cold.

The manufacturers advise changing the lancet needle every time. I change mine when I remember or if it gets a bit blunt. I have never had an infection as a result of doing that, nor have I ever heard of it happening from the people I talk to on the web. You do what you are comfortable with, subject to doctor's orders.

The best advice I received from any source, professional or otherwise, after I was diagnosed with type 2 diabetes was written by a lady named Jennifer. I first met her in cyber-space posting on the alt.support.diabetes usenet group where she regularly greeted newly diagnosed people with the advice I repeat below. It still appears as "Jennifer's Information for the Newly Diagnosed" on the alt.support.diabetes home page at http://www.alt-support-diabetes.org/new.php and has now been repeated on many other web-sites. Some years ago she graciously gave me permission to spread it far and wide. I have been doing that ever since.

Jennifer's Information for the Newly Diagnosed

Sounds like you're planning a move to take control of your diabetes... good for you.

There is so much to absorb... you do not have to rush into anything. Begin by using your best weapon in this war, your meter. You won't keel over today, you have time to experiment, test, learn, test and figure out just how your body and this disease are getting along. The most important thing you can do to learn about yourself and diabetes is test test test.

The single biggest question a diabetic has to answer is:

What do I eat?

Unfortunately, the answer is pretty confusing. What confounds us all is the fact that different diabetics can get great results on wildly different food plans. Some of us here achieve great blood glucose control eating a high complex carbohydrate diet. Others find that anything over 75 - 100g of carbohydrates a day is too much. Still others are somewhere in between.

At the beginning all of us felt frustrated. We wanted to be handed THE way to eat, to ensure our continued health. But we all learned that there is no one way. Each of us had to find our own path, using the experience of those that went before, but still having to discover for ourselves how OUR bodies and this disease were coexisting. Ask questions, but remember each of us discovered on our own what works best for us. You can use our experiences as jumping off points, but eventually you'll work up a successful plan that is yours alone.

What you are looking to discover is how different foods affect you. As I am sure you have read, carbohydrates (sugars, wheat, rice... the things our Grandmas called "starches") raise blood sugars the most rapidly. Protein and fat do raise them, but not as high and much more slowly... so if you're a T2, generally the insulin your body still makes may take care of the rise.

You might want to try some experiments.

First: Eat whatever you have been currently eating... but

write it all down.
Test yourself at the following times:

Upon waking (fasting)
1 hour after each meal
2 hours after each meal
At bedtime

That means 8 x each day. What you will discover by this is how long after a meal your highest reading comes... and how fast you return to "normal". Also, you may see that a meal that included bread, fruit or other carbohydrates gives you a higher reading.

Then for the next few days, try to curb your carbohydrates. Eliminate breads, cereals, rice, beans, any wheat products, potato, corn, fruit... get all your carbohydrates from veggies. Test at the same schedule above.

If you try this for a few days, you may find some pretty good readings. It is worth a few days to discover. Eventually you can slowly add back carbohydrates until you see them affecting your meter. The thing about this disease... though we share much in common and we need to follow certain guidelines... in the end, each of our bodies dictate our treatment and our success.

The closer we get to non-diabetic numbers, the greater chance we have of avoiding horrible complications. The key here is AIM... I know that everyone is at a different point in their disease... and it is progressive. But, if we aim for the best numbers and do our best, we give ourselves the best shot at health we have got. That is all we can do.

Here's my opinion on what numbers to aim for, they are non-diabetic numbers.

Fasting	*under 110*
One hour after meals	*under 140*
Two hours after meals	*under 120*

or for those in the mmol parts of the world:

Fasting	*under 6*
One hour after meals	*under 8*
Two hours after meals	*under 6.5*

Recent studies have indicated that the most important numbers are your "after meal" numbers. They may be the most indicative of future complications, especially heart problems.

Listen to your doctor, but you are the leader of your diabetic care team. While his /her advice is learned, it is not absolute. You will end up knowing much more about your body and how it is handling diabetes than your doctor will. Your meter is your best weapon.

Just remember, we're not in a race or a competition with anyone but ourselves... Play around with your food plan... TEST TEST TEST. Learn what foods cause spikes, what foods cause cravings... Use your body as a science experiment.

You'll read about a lot of different ways people use to

control their diabetes... Many are diametrically opposed. After awhile you'll learn that there is no one size fits all around here. Take some time to experiment and you'll soon discover the plan that works for you.

Best of luck!

Jennifer.

As an engineer, when I read that, it made sense immediately. So simple, yet so powerful. And it has certainly worked for me.

I used Jennifer's advice to gain control of my numbers fairly quickly. Once I understood it I did not mess about and I used a lot of test strips in those early days. I fairly rapidly achieved the goals she set and I realised that I could do better.

At the time, despite their poor advice on carbohydrates and rather loose guidelines for blood glucose targets, the ADA recommended something that stuck in my mind: "Keeping your blood glucose as close to normal as possible helps you feel better and reduces the risk of long-term complications of diabetes." That sounded logical to me so eventually I changed Jennifer's goals for myself to my present goals of:

Fasting	under 100
One hour after meals	under 120
Two hours after meals	under 100

or for those in the mmol parts of the world:

Fasting   under 5.5
One hour after meals   under 6.5
Two hours after meals   under 5.5

Over time you will choose new targets for yourself when you find a comfortable balance between your diabetes management goals and your lifestyle needs.

I also changed the after-meal testing times from one and two hours to my peak timing. See Chapter 6, Testing, Testing, for more detail on that.

I live in a country that uses Millimoles per litre, or mmol/L, as the units for measurement of blood glucose and cholesterol levels. Canada, the United Kingdom and many other countries also use those units. Unfortunately, most of the books on Type 2 diabetes are published in the USA, which is also where the most active diabetes forums are based. The USA uses a quite different system of units: milligrams per decilitre (mg/dL), for exactly the same blood tests.

I have not the faintest idea why that is the case, but for those who wish to read about or discuss diabetes beyond their own borders it can be very useful to be able to convert from one to the other.

Cholesterol or Lipids

To convert from mmol/L to mg/dl for cholesterol or lipids panels including Total Cholesterol (TC), LDL, HDL or VLDL divide by 0.0259 or multiply by 38.6. For a quick estimate multiply by 40.

For Triglycerides divide by 0.0113 or multiply by 88.5. For a quick estimate multiply by 90.

Lipids ratios are mentioned in several papers discussing their relevance to cardiac risk and insulin resistance; remember to use conversions before applying US numbers. For example, some papers recommend that the triglycerides/HDL ratio should be under 1:1.3 when using mmol/L units; the US mg/dL equivalent is to be under 1:3.0.

The Friedewald Formula, used to calculate a cholesterol component such as LDL when only the others were measured, is as follows:

Using mg/dL

Total Cholesterol = LDL + HDL + triglycerides/5

Using mmol/L

Total Cholesterol = LDL + HDL + triglycerides/2.18

Blood Glucose

The conversion can be done either by multiplying by 18 or divide by .0555 if you want to be really accurate. The exact multiplier is 18.018. When accuracy is not critical, using a multiplier of 20 can be quick and useful. To be honest, as most meters have tolerances significantly greater than +/- 5%, trying for exact conversion accuracy is a waste of time in my opinion.

A list of the units used around the world is available at DiabetesExplained.com. Their url is http://www.diabetesexplained.com/country-units.html

Quick Blood Glucose Conversion Table

mg/dL	mmol/L	mmol/L	mg/dL
60	3.3	3.5	63
70	3.9	4	72
80	4.4	4.5	81
90	5.0	5	90
100	5.6	5.5	99
110	6.1	6	108
120	6.7	6.5	117
130	7.2	7	126
140	7.8	7.5	135
150	8.3	8	144
160	8.9	8.5	153
170	9.4	9	162
180	10.0	9.5	171
190	10.5	10	180
200	11.1	11	198
250	13.9	15	270
300	16.7	20	360
400	22.2	25	450

For those who wish to get into the nitty-gritty of the science and logic supporting the ideas in this book, the books below are well worth reading. I treat the information available from all sources about diabetes as a smorgasbord; I take what makes sense to me and works for me, and leave what does not. I benefited most from Gretchen Becker's book. Bernstein also has a wealth of good ideas although his dietary ideas may be a little strict for some. I was lucky to learn personally from Jenny Ruhl when she was a regular contributor on alt.support.diabetes. Since then she has published her own book; it is very readable and Jenny also has a wealth of useful and practical information well supported by scientific cites.

These are available from your library, good bookstore or Amazon.

The First Year, Type 2 Diabetes, An Essential Guide for the Newly Diagnosed. Author: Gretchen Becker. ISBN-13: 978-1569245460

Dr. Bernstein's Diabetes Solution, Revised and Updated, by Richard K, Bernstein, M.D., ISBN-13: 978-0316167161

Blood Sugar 101, What They Don't Tell you about Diabetes, by Jenny Ruhl, ISBN-13: 978-0964711617.

Magazines and cook books

All the magazines I have read on diabetes were only suitable for one thing and they were too glossy to be much use for that. The same applies to all "Diabetes" recipe books and magazines. If you need a recipe book, look for a low-carbohydrate recipe book, not a diabetes recipe book.

Links

This is not an exhaustive list, but some, like Mendosa, have links to many others. Those which require registration have never sent me a spam or unwanted promotional emails. My own blog is "Type 2 Diabetes, A Personal Journey" at:
http://loraldiabetes.blogspot.com/

Please note that although there is a lot of good information on many of these sites I do not necessarily agree with all, or any, of the information presented. Also be aware that the websites listed in this book may change without notice.

General links

Jennifer's "Test, Test, Test":
http://www.alt-support-diabetes.org/new.php

alt.support.diabetes home page:
http://www.alt-support-diabetes.org/index.php

The misc.health.diabetes FAQs:
http://www.faqs.org/faqs/diabetes/

dLife:
http://www.dlife.com/

David Mendosa:
http://www.mendosa.com/

Jenny (Janet) Ruhl:
Blood Sugar 101: http://www.phlaunt.com/diabetes
Blog: http://diabetesupdate.blogspot.com/

Joslin:
http://joslin.org/

The AACE:
http://www.aace.com/index.php

The ADA:
http://www.diabetes.org/

Diabetes Australia:
http://www.diabetesaustralia.com.au/en/

Diabetes UK:
http://www.diabetes.org.uk/home.htm

National Institute of Diabetes and Digestive and Kidney Diseases (NIDDK):
http://diabetes.niddk.nih.gov/

UK Prospective Diabetes Study (Type 2):
http://www.dtu.ox.ac.uk/index.php

Diabetes Control and Complications Trial (DCCT) (Type 1):
http://diabetes.niddk.nih.gov/dm/pubs/control/

Medical searchers, journals and similar

Highwire:
http://highwire.stanford.edu/

Medscape (registration required):
http://www.medscape.com/medscapetoday

Google Scholar:
http://scholar.google.com/advanced_scholar_search

Heart:
http://www.theheart.org/

New England Journal of Medicine
http://www.nejm.org/

Journal of the American Medical Association
http://jama.ama-assn.org/

Present Diabetes, an education site
www.presentdiabetes.com/

Diabetes in Control
http://www.diabetesincontrol.com/

Discussion Groups on the Web

Yahoo Diabetes World:
http://health.groups.yahoo.com/group/diabetesworld/

ADA Discussions (previously ADA Forums):
http://connect.diabetes.org/discussions

dLife Forum:
http://www.dlife.com/diabetes-forum/

Diabetes Support Forum UK:
http://www.diabetes-support.org.uk/

Diabetes Forum UK:
http://diabetesforum.org.uk/

Usenet Newsgroups

Get ready for unmoderated anarchy. There are some very nice and very knowledgeable diabetics on usenet if you don a flame-proof suit and wade through the spam, kooks and nasty people:

alt.support.diabetes
alt.support.diabetes.uk
misc.health.diabetes
alt.food.diabetic

One of the consequences of diagnosis with diabetes is a need to plan if we intend to travel long distances. The security needs for modern air travel have created additional difficulties but even road trips require planning.

AIR TRAVEL

Travel by air has become a bit more complicated since 9/11. I was travelling through the USA in March 2003 when the Iraq war started. Security went nuts and within a week we missed a flight from St Louis to Atlanta because we spent over two hours in security. The American Transportation Security Administration (TSA) took a long time to find a way to secure air travel without grossly inconveniencing passengers. However, after the initial over-reaction things have settled a bit now.

Hypo protection

I carry jelly beans for the possibility of lows. In the USA Smarties can also serve that purpose. They are simple, not bulky and easily fit in a pocket or purse. Another advantage is that they should cause no problems with security or food quarantine inspectors. Although it is a long time since my last hypo, I do not want to find I am having my next one on a plane with no suitable food handy.

Mid Air Snacks

Making some snacks up in advance is best because you can choose exactly what they are. You are not restricted to the over-priced limited range available at the airport or on the plane. I usually make up a small sealed plastic container of mixed nuts and raisins. It keeps well, can be kept in a pocket or purse for a quick nibble to stave off hunger and gives a good mix of protein, fats and carbohydrate. It also does not cause any problems getting through airport security, which can be just as important these days. If that is not possible, I seek out something suitable in the airside shops. I look for foods such as beef jerky (check the carbohydrate count), nuts, cheese-'n-crackers or similar. Not for meals, but for those times when you need something to nibble during a long flight. I do not try for very low carbohydrate, instead I usually have a balanced mix of carbohydrates, protein and fat including about 5-10 gms carbohydrate in a snack.

I never go on a flight without sufficient for two or three snacks in my carry-on. It may be scheduled as a one-hour hop. After the first time you have waited three hours in the gate lounge and then sat in a delayed plane on the taxi-way for several hours without food, air-conditioning or information, you realise that travelling in those conditions without snacks is not wise. It may only ever happen to you once, but that will be too often if you do not have food available every few hours.

In-flight Meals

This is becoming a hypothetical subject, but there are still a diminishing number of airlines that provide meals in cattle class.

Never, ever, ring in advance to advise that you have diabetes and wish to have a "diabetic" meal. If you do, be ready to eat a meal that will commence with a bread roll, followed by a main of low fat starch, with sides of starch, washed down with fruit juice, followed by a piece of fruit and a dessert of low-sugar rice pudding or similar.

Instead, I have a standard procedure. I wait until the initial boarding rush is over and I can catch the attention of the steward. I advise the steward that I have diabetes that I manage with a strict diet. Then I patiently nod and smile through the set "you should have advised us in advance so we could have provided a special diabetic meal for you". I apologise for not doing so and request a look at the menu of the day. I then choose the least bad choice. Failure to do this means you are risking no choice at all when they run out of the beef casserole and you find that pasta and rice is the only choice left. On two notable occasions, when there were no remotely acceptable choices, the senior steward suggested that I might prefer something from the business class menu. You get a different class of service on Qantas and Air New

Zealand.

For longer flights I carry an insulated soft cooler pack with me as a carry-on. It doubles as my carry-on for medications and other things I need to get at quickly. Most airlines will allow something like that as a second carry-on, but check if your airline has a one-bag limit.

I often prepare a salad the night before, usually with some cold cuts or similar, and pack it in an appropriate small plastic lunch container. The dry food will get through the TSA security, but liquids won't. I have not tried a freezer brick through security since the rules on liquids changed; instead I suggest that you transfer the food from the fridge to the cooler pack as late as possible. After passing through security buy a cold drink which can also act as a cooler for the insulated section. If you do not want to prepare in advance you can nearly always buy a prepared salad or jerky or something similar on the over-priced "air" side of security.

This brochure on air travel from the ADA notes that drinks for diabetics are now allowed through security based on the doctor's letter:
Fact Sheet: Air Travel and Diabetes:
http://www.diabetes.org/assets/pdfs/know-your-rights/public-accommodations/fact-sheet-tsa.pdf

I was able to get a diet soda through security at Noumea, New Caledonia, by producing evidence of my diagnosis, but I would not count on it elsewhere. If you are departing a foreign country retain some local currency just in case you need to buy your cans or bottles after the security check. On board, I have never travelled on an airline that did not provide water or diet soda on demand, sometimes free.

Medications and Diabetes Supplies

When I fly I always carry a letter from my doctor listing my ailments and medications. I have rarely needed that letter, but on those rare occasions it saved me a lot of stress and hassle.

For diabetes supplies read the current rules on the TSA web-site. They apply to all US airports and many overseas airports also use them as a general guide. Here are the present urls:

Travellers with Disabilities and Medical Conditions
http://www.tsa.gov/travelers/airtravel/specialneeds/in dex.shtm

Hidden Disabilities (including diabetes)
http://www.tsa.gov/travelers/airtravel/specialneeds/e ditorial_1374.shtm#3

3-1-1 for carry-ons http://www.tsa.gov/311/index.shtm

If the urls have changed by the time you read this you should be able to find the pages by starting at the home page, http://www.tsa.gov/index.shtm, and using those titles for a search

Note that the 3-1-1 gels and liquids rule is eased for medications. They do not need to go in that quart zip-loc bag. For the specific rules go to the "Travellers with Disabilities and Medical Conditions" site and scroll down to: "Additionally, we are continuing to permit prescription liquid medications and other liquids needed by persons with disabilities and medical conditions" and subsequent paragraphs. That was a very useful tip explained to me by the TSA supervisor at DFW. It helped that I had my letter from my doctor, but items not on the doc's list such as mosquito repellent, antiseptic and similar were also allowed.

ROAD TRIPS

When possible I prepare snacks as I do for an air trip and carry the cooler pack on board. That gets a lot of use in the car because there will always be a bottle or two of diet soft drinks, a bottle of wine and some cheese and crackers or similar. I add a couple of freezer bricks to keep things cold and fresh. Each night I put one of those in the room fridge, if it has one, or ask the hotel staff to keep it in the restaurant freezer. I have never had that request rejected but I have occasionally forgotten to collect it in the morning. I also store small containers of olive oil for salad dressing or cooking oil, vinegar, salt and pepper in the side pockets.

Meals on the Road

I have given some general tips in the Eating Out and Breakfasts chapters. However, there are a couple of other tricks I use when I am on the road.

You do not have to go to the lengths I do; treat my ideas like a smorgasbord – choose what suits you, leave what does not.

I look for diners and "Mom and Pop" restaurants. The type of place where I can get bacon and eggs for breakfast, or they will listen when I ask them to hold the fries and double the salad. I have often found their food to be at least as good as hotel restaurants. They may lack in ambience and the decor may need some paint or paper, but I also met lots of nice people to chat to in those diners in far corners of the world. I didn't meet many to chat to in sterile hotels or high-class restaurants, although I must admit I eat in those less often.

If the accommodation I am using has cooking facilities I always prefer to cook my own simple breakfasts. While on the road it is easy to pick up some ham or bacon, eggs, maybe an onion, mushrooms, cheese (or whatever you like) to cook bacon and eggs or make a simple omelette or scrambled eggs in the morning.

As I usually travel for weeks or months at a time and many hotels do not have cooking facilities I often also carry a small bag with a small electric skillet and a few cooking utensils with me. Not much, usually a couple of plates and bowls, some basic cutlery and tools for the skillet. It does not take much effort to whip up a quick omelette or bacon and eggs in the morning, and there isn't much to clean up. The only difficulty is a need to be careful not to set off the hotel room's smoke detectors.

RECIPES

Recipes: Keeping it Simple

The recipes that follow are basic examples to show that cooking for better health does not need to be complicated or difficult. I have cooked or prepared all of these many times.

In all of my recipes the quantities are extremely flexible and subject to the foods that happen to be in the fridge and pantry at the time. Cooking should not add stress to your day. For example, I often use highly precise Australian measurements such as a "slurp" or a "smidgin" or a "grating". Use your imagination.

My flexible ingredients mean that the nutrition tables I provide are only intended as a broad guide. You should always test after your meal when you try any new recipe to see if it is right for you.

Please experiment and develop your own favourites. Every recipe is a base, add what you like that you think will work. However, it is usually wise to try the recipe as written the first time.

Use any of the blank pages to add your own notes for personal variations and extensions of these recipes.

Bon appetit.

Stir Fry and Salad Mix

You have done the right thing and bought a wider variety of vegetables. But now you are running out of ideas on how to use them. I know what that is like. Steamed vegetables can get fairly boring fairly quickly. It is even worse if you boil them to a mush; apart from having no texture or flavour many of the good vitamins will disappear down the drain with the water you boiled them in.

Sometimes you just don't feel like doing the work of scrubbing, peeling and preparing vegetables when all you want is a quick lunch or a light dinner. I developed this idea as a way of always having something ready in the fridge for a quick salad or a stir-fry with minimal preparation at cooking or meal preparation time. Like most of my small repertoire of recipes this can be prepared when time is available so that meal time can be quick and easy.

Basic Mix

1 medium onion, sliced
1 cup coarsely chopped cabbage (any type)
1 diced carrot
1 cup capsicum (bell pepper), preferably yellow
A few stalks of chopped celery

Options

Add all or any of these, but at least three or four different ingredients in addition to the basic mix. Measurements, unless stated otherwise, are between a half-cup and a cup. Corn and beans are subject to their affect on your after-meal **blood glucose** levels, but as this is spread across multiple serves you'll find they should not be a problem. Chop or dice as appropriate.

Red or Green Capsicum (bell pepper)
Cauliflower florettes and chopped stems
Broccoli Florettes and chopped stems
Green Peas
Green (string) beans
Snow (snap) peas
½ cup sweet corn kernels
½ cup cooked kidney beans
Assorted cooked other beans
Raw asparagus
Bok Choi
Scallions or eschallottes
Leeks

Add or substitute anything else I may have forgotten that you like or that is in season in your district. After preparation, cover the bowl and store it in the fridge. It should keep fresh and crisp for several days.

Use this as a general purpose base for stir-fries or simply add your favourite dressing to it for a quick salad. For a stir-fry I often use it just as it is, but sometimes I fry some chopped onion, ginger and garlic, then the sliced meat or fish before adding the mix. I add spices or sauce and water at the appropriate time as it cooks in the wok.

As a salad use a cup or two per person as a serve. You can also add things such as lettuce, tomato, avocado, or diced cheddar at serving time for a salad but do not put them in the mix for storage because they will not keep well. Add cold cuts or ham, or a vegetarian equivalent, for protein at serving time. One of my favourite quick lunches is to add a small can of tuna to a large cup of the salad mix and mix in a couple of tablespoons of whole-egg mayonnaise.

Simple Salad Dressing

In a small bottle with a cap mix four tablespoons of extra virgin olive oil, one tablespoon of balsamic vinegar, one tablespoon of white vinegar, a small chopped clove of garlic, a touch of hot chilli to taste, some chopped garden herbs (basil, thyme, rosemary, mint, whatever are your favourites); shake well and add lightly to the salad. It will keep for a long time in the fridge. Let it warm up to room temperature before using it so that the oil will become fully liquid again.

Hearty Vegetable Soup

The advantage of this recipe is that it is simple and totally flexible. The recipe creates 10-12 large (320ml) serves of soup from ¾ hour's preparation and an hour's simmering. After cooking and cooling I store the results in single-serve containers in the freezer. This would be my lunch two or three days a week; straight from the freezer via the microwave.

I have given an example of the ingredients in a batch I cooked recently. However, you should use your favourite or seasonal vegetables. The only proviso is that you try to include slightly more watery or green vegetables than root vegetables. That gives a wider mix of vitamins and flavours and reduces the carbohydrates. The nutrition table is based on my choices in the list below.

Ingredients

1 can of peeled tomatoes
3 tablespoons of Pearl Barley
1 medium onion
½ of one capsicum (bell pepper)
1 large carrot
1 medium potato
A few stalks of celery
1 large cup of cabbage
1 large cup of broccoli chunks – including the stem

Method

Half-fill two large pots with water and bring them to the boil; reduce to a simmer. I use a two-litre (roughly half-gallon) pot for my "blender pot" and one twice that size for my "main pot".

Blender pot preparation

Add the can of tomatoes and bring it to the simmer. As you later prepare vegetables, scrub and wash them thoroughly first and then put any peels, celery tops, carrot ends, cabbage cores etc into the blender pot. I waste nothing edible.

A tip for those who cook for fussy eaters such as children or spouses with pet aversions to certain vegetables. Put all of the vegetables they "won't eat" in the blender pot. But never let the diners see the contents of that pot until you have reached the stage where it is a puree.

Main pot preparation

Add a bone from a ham or a leftover roast joint or similar to the main pot to become part of the stock base. Personally, I like the little bits of stewed meat that leave the bone, but if you do not like the meat scraps becoming part of the soup do that separately in advance and strain the liquid into the main pot. Whenever we have a lamb or pork roast, or buy a new ham for freezing chunks, the next free afternoon is soup-making time. Or just add a few stock cubes or commercial stock. Then add the pearl barley and bring the pot to the simmer.

Prepare the vegetables. Roughly chop or dice the vegetables as you like them. Add the neatest chunks or pieces to the main pot and all the peels and scrappy bits to the blender pot.

Crush a couple of cloves of garlic and add to the blender pot. Ensure there is adequate water in both pots to let them simmer safely for at least an hour. Check and stir occasionally, top up the water if necessary, but allow space in the main pot for the two to be combined at the finish. The hour, which is a minimum, not a maximum is needed for the barley to fully cook and the bone to add its flavour.

Remove the blender pot from the heat. When it is cool enough to use your stick blender, blend it to a puree and stir that into the main pot after removing the bone from that pot.

I like my soup chunky, but if you prefer a thicker, less chunky soup, use the stick blender to achieve your desired consistency. If you like it thinner, add some boiling water and let it simmer again for a few minutes. Adjust seasoning (salt and pepper) to taste.

When it has cooled sufficiently fill single-serve individual freezer containers with the soup and store them for future use. When you want a quick and simple lunch, decant the container into a soup bowl (I run it under a tap to loosen it) and zap it in the microwave. If you take lunch to work, heat it in the morning and take it in a wide-mouth thermos.

Nutrition Table

This will vary depending on things like the fat on the soup bone and the proportion of root vegetables and barley. The version I make is approximately as follows, dividing into ten large serves:

Calories	60
Kilojoules	250
Protein	2 gm
Total Fat	<1 gm
Carbohydrate	12 gm
Fibre	3 gm

Beef Burgundy

I often add copious quantities of mushrooms or carrot or celery to this one, depending on what's in the larder.

Ingredients

1kg (2 ½ lb) Stewing steak. Use any cheap cut of beef. The cheaper the cut, the longer you cook it.

125 gm (1/4 lb) Bacon
1 medium onion
2 cloves garlic
1 or 2 tablespoons plain flour or 1 teaspoon guar gum
Black pepper
Nutmeg
Salt
Olive oil
One bottle of red wine

Method

Chop the bacon roughly, slice the onion into rings and crush the garlic. Sauté the bacon, onion and garlic in a tablespoon of the oil in a heavy skillet or pot over moderate heat until the onion is transparent, then remove it from the skillet and set it aside temporarily. If you are trying to lose weight and the fat worries you, drain it on kitchen paper. I don't bother.

Remove as much fat and gristle as you reasonably can from the beef. Roughly cut it into chunks, about 2 cm (3/4") cubes. I cut my pieces a little smaller than most cooks because this is one of my favourite breakfast stews and smaller pieces seem more palatable at breakfast time. Add a little more oil to the skillet and quickly fry the beef over high heat in small batches until browned and sealed, but not cooked. Set the meat aside in a casserole dish that has an appropriate cover.

Return the bacon, onion and garlic to the skillet and mix in a tablespoon of flour. Stir while cooking lightly, brown but do not burn. Guar gum can be used as a carbohydrate-free thickener but you will need to experiment to get the quantity and method right; about a level teaspoon in this recipe. I prefer flour in this recipe, as the flavour seems better and the tablespoon is spread across six serves. Flour also seems to combine better with the wine.

Add a large glass of red wine and stir while cooking until the sauce thickens. If the sauce is too thick, add a little more wine or water until the consistency is thick but pourable and not gluey. If it is too thin, add a little flour to a little water, stir the lumps out, and add it to the sauce. Add freshly ground black pepper, a good grating of nutmeg and a little salt to taste.

Add the sauce to the meat in the casserole dish, cover and place in a slow (170c, 340F) oven for an hour and a half or longer if a cheap cut was used. Check and stir, cook for another half-hour, then turn the oven off but leave it in the oven for another half-hour.

The cook is entitled to drink some of the remaining wine while awaiting completion of the cooking process. Of course, you may drink the rest at dinner.

Serve as it is, or with brown or basmati rice if you can handle the carbohydrates. Serves 4 - 8, depending on serve size and accompaniments. I turn it into lots of small breakfasts, by freezing small individual serves.

Nutrition Table

Based on six serves using flour for thickener:

Calories	475
Kilojoules	1990
Protein	28 gm
Total Fat	36 gm
Carbohydrate	6 gm
Fibre	1 gm

Cheesy Guacamole Dip

Ingredients

Chopped ingredients are to the texture you like. I like some lumps and crunchy bits, but if you do not, then chop them finely.

1 ripe avocado
¼ cup finely chopped celery
¼ cup chopped onion
¼ cup chopped red capsicum (bell pepper)
1 chopped hot chilli pepper (to your taste, or chilli flakes)
½ minced clove of garlic
30g chopped cheddar cheese
30g light Philadelphia or ricotta or cottage cheese
2 teaspoons grated parmesan
A large squeeze of lemon or lime juice - essential for longer life in the fridge
1/2 tsp minced/grated ginger (optional)
Salt and pepper to taste

All ingredients are extremely approximate and depend on what is in the fridge. For that reason I have not included a nutrition table.

Peel the avocado, mix the flesh with all the dry ingredients and then add the lemon juice. Adjust dryness with olive or peanut oil if necessary until a smooth paste is obtained.

If you are using a food processor add the solid vegetable ingredients last and process very briefly to retain some texture.

Serve this with slices of carrot, celery or similar for dipping. Thin low fat crackers may be OK depending on your carbohydrate requirements.

This is low in carbohydrates subject to whether you use crackers for dipping. The fat content depends on proportions of full-fat and low fat cheeses. Check your **blood glucose level** at one hour; mine is usually good after this.

Use it to fill that "gotta have something" gap between meals.

Napoli Sauce

My apologies to anyone of Italian extraction - I know it is not like Momma used to make.

I cook this sauce up in bulk and use it in various other recipes like spaghetti bolognese, stuffed mushrooms, minimal-carbohydrate pizzas etc. I also like it as a low-carbohydrate sugar-free alternative to ketchup on steak, hamburgers and other cooked meats.

It will keep for a few days in the fridge, but I usually freeze it in two ways. About half of a bulk lot I freeze as ice cubes which I then transfer to an old ice-cream container in the freezer for ready use. Then I can defrost the number necessary without waste, as I often cook for one. The remainder I freeze in larger 1 or 2 cup serves in plastic containers for use as needed. I always have a thawed one in the fridge for ready use as a ketchup or sauce.

Vary the ingredients, particularly herbs, to your own taste. However, it may be best to follow the recipe with a small test try first.

Ingredients

1 can (about 400g or 14 oz) peeled tomatoes, or fresh equivalent
1 medium onion, chopped
1/4 cup tomato paste (optional)

1 clove of garlic, minced
Olive oil
Cracked black pepper to taste
Salt to taste
1 teaspoon of dried basil or a few chopped leaves

If you like other herbs such as oregano, thyme etc, just adjust to your taste, but basil is basic to the recipe.

Method

Sweat the chopped onion in a large pot over medium heat until translucent but not brown. Use a little olive oil to prevent sticking to the pot.

Add the minced garlic and cook until also translucent.

Chop the tomatoes and add them to the pot with their juice. For large quantities drain the liquid into the onion mix and use a processor for the solids in batches. Or, if you have a stick blender, blend it in the pot - it does not need to be a puree, I prefer some texture. The tomatoes will break down further as they cook.

Add the basil and any other herbs and bring the mix to a slow covered simmer. Allow it to simmer for at least an hour, longer if possible, until the tomato breaks down and the onion seems to almost disappear.

Check and stir occasionally to prevent sticking; add a

little water if the mixture gets too thick. When the sauce is cooked it should be thicker but still liquid and pourable. Adjust seasoning near the end.

For a richer, thicker sauce add the tomato paste towards the finish and cook while stirring until it is cooked in. If you add it too early you will need to watch more closely for sticking.

Bulk cooking

I just multiply; usually I cook about six cans worth. How much you cook depends on the size of your saucepan or cooker and your storage and freezing facilities. As you increase the quantity you may need to adjust the onion, garlic and basil quantities down a little in proportion.

Nutrition Table.

Per cup. The total fat content is from the olive oil.

Calories	140
Kilojoules	590
Protein	2.5 gm
Total Fat	7 gm
Carbohydrate	18 gm
Fibre	9.5 gm

Sweet Curry

This curry has a surprisingly low carbohydrate count for the sweet taste of the sauce.

Ingredients

All measures and weights are very approximate. Tablespoons are level, not heaped.

2 tablespoons olive oil
600gm (1½ lb) chuck steak
1 onion
1 clove garlic
1 cooking apple
Juice ½ lemon
30gm (1oz) sultanas or raisins
2 **tablespoons** curry powder
1 **tablespoon** flour
1 **tablespoon** chutney
300 ml (1/2 pint) stock or water and stock cube.

Method

Trim fat and gristle and cut the meat into rough cubes of 2cm or 3/4".

Sear the meat in one tablespoon of olive oil in a medium saucepan and transfer to the casserole pot when browned.

Sauté the onion in the pan juices, add a little more oil if necessary. When the onions are translucent, add the chopped garlic and the peeled and roughly diced apple. Stir in first the curry powder, then the flour and then add the stock.

Bring to the boil, add the chutney, lemon juice and raisins and simmer for five minutes.

Add the sauce to the browned meat in the casserole pot. Cover and cook in a slow oven (150C, 300F) for two hours. Stir occasionally; adjust liquid by adding a smidgin of water if necessary. Turn the oven off 30 minutes before serving and leave it in the cooling oven.

Serve with a side salad if you are watching the carbohydrates, with steamed rice if you're not. I can handle a heaped tablespoon of rice with it in the evening; let your meter decide. Sometimes I add some chopped carrots or celery in the sauce, but keep an eye on the carbohydrates if you add carrot. Serves 4.

Nutrition Table (without rice):

Calories	320
Kilojoules	1340
Protein	24 gm
Total Fat	17 gm
Carbohydrate	18 gm
Fibre	3 gm

Breakfast Stew

I make this up every month or two and use the results for breakfast once or twice a week. All measurements are approximate; it is one of those "make it up as you go along" type of dishes. The main thing is to not add too many high-carbohydrate vegetables to it; no spuds for example. Carrots are OK for me but they do spike some people, so adjust to suit yourself. Replace them with something like cabbage or capsicum or any non-starchy vegetable you like in season.

Ingredients

1.5-2kg (3.5-4lbs) approx of stewing beef or lamb
2 cups celery, chopped
2 large carrots, sliced
1 medium/large onion, chopped
4 cloves garlic, minced or crushed
1 rasher or 4 strips of bacon, chopped
Chopped herbs to your taste; I use basil, mint and thyme.

Method

In a large frying pan or wok fry the onions, garlic and chopped bacon in a little olive oil until the onion is starting to lightly brown. Add the celery, carrots and herbs and cook until the vegetables have started to "sweat" but are not fully cooked. Transfer to a bowl temporarily.

Trim the beef of fat and gristle and cut it into cubes of 1-2cm, or 1/2"-3/4". Fry the meat on high heat in a little olive oil in the same pan, in small batches, until they are sealed and brown but not cooked. Transfer to an appropriate sized casserole container for your oven. Do not fry too much at once or the meat will release too much liquid and not brown correctly.

When all the meat has been fried and is in the casserole container, return the reserved vegetables to the pan and sprinkle a teaspoon of guar gum over them. Mix that well and add a cup or two of dry red wine to de-glaze the pan. Bring the mixture to the boil, simmer for a couple of minutes, then pour the vegetable mix over the meat.

Mix and then add sufficient stock (or water and stock cubes) so that the result will be just enough to cover the mixture of meat and vegetables. Press down the mixture with a large spoon so that the liquid just covers the meats.

Cook in a 140-160C (285-320F) oven for about 90 minutes (longer if it is a cheap cut of meat) and leave it in the oven another 30 minutes after you turn off the heat. About half-way through, season with salt and pepper to your taste.

I also add a few sliced mushrooms to the mix sometimes.

Let it cool in the fridge overnight. Put 7-10 small

individual serves in plastic containers in the freezer. When you want a quick no-fuss breakfast decant it into a bowl, zap it in the microwave while making your coffee or having your shower - and presto - breakfast.

Nutrition Table

Based on those ingredients and 8 serves, this is an approximate nutrition breakdown:

Calories	400
Kilojoules	1675
Protein	38 gm
Total Fat	20 gm
Carbohydrate	6 gm
Fibre	2 gm

Psyllium, Fibre, Muesli and Nuts

I gradually cut the starchy and high GI carbohydrates in my daily menu significantly as I changed my menu using feedback from my meter.

I replaced them with other vegetables but on analysis I decided that I needed to add some fibre back into my menu. After some investigation I found that the most readily available supplement to do that was psyllium husk; a food that is 80-85% dietary fibre. If you do a little searching on psyllium you will find a lot of scientific papers on its various benefits. However, it is not easy to eat the stuff directly. That is why commercially available forms such as Metamucil have other flavours and ingredients added to make them palatable.

Separate to that, I also found that I could eat more carbohydrates in the evening and that a small bowl of muesli at bedtime helped with my dawn effect numbers in the morning. Additionally, I try to eat some nuts regularly as part of my menu.

As a result of all those different factors I gradually developed this simple recipe for my bedtime snack. I eat this three or four times a week. One other beneficial side effect is excellent morning regularity.

Ingredients

One 750gm or 1 Kg (1 1/2 to 2 lbs) pack of Muesli from the supermarket. For those who have not eaten Muesli, it is usually a mix of rolled oats, other grains, dried fruits and similar food. It is high in whole grains and fruits, so it is high in carbohydrates but also high in fibre. The brand I buy is usually about 65% carbohydrate and 10-14% fibre.

400-500 gms of mixed nuts, roasted but not salted. My usual mix is brazils, walnuts, almonds, cashews; I vary it occasionally with pecans or other real nuts. No peanuts.

200-250gm psyllium husks.

The result is roughly a 4:2:1 ratio of Muesli to nuts to psyllium.

Method

I chop the nuts coarsely in a food processor, but not to the point where they are a powder. I like the crunch when I eat them. Then I just mix all the ingredients together and store them in a large air-tight container.

Using the Mix

Test to see what portion size and time of day is best for you. I cannot eat this at breakfast time; possibly you can. At bedtime I put two or three tablespoons of the mix in a bowl and cover it with enough whole milk to wet it. I experimented to find the quantity needed to overcome the psyllium husk's tendency to set the mix solid.

Occasionally I use water instead of milk, or a combination of both.

Nutrition Table

For my most recent mix I worked out the actual numbers (US style, subtract fibre) for a 40gm serve with 100ml whole milk. These numbers will vary according to your muesli ingredients and choice of nuts.

Calories	220
Kilojoules	920
Protein	8 gm
Total Fat	12 gm
Carbohydrate	27 gm
Fibre	8.5 gm

Stuffed Mushrooms

Breakfast for one, low carbohydrate.

Ingredients

1 small onion
1 very large mushroom (saucer sized) or two or three medium to large mushrooms
2 or 3 tablespoons of Napoli Sauce or chopped canned tomatoes
Grated or sliced Cheddar
Grated parmesan cheese
Olive or canola oil for cooking.
Salt, grated black pepper and nutmeg to taste

Skillet method.

I use a 6" cast-iron skillet.

Remove, but do not discard, the stalks from the mushrooms, peel the mushrooms if appropriate.

Pre-heat the skillet and your grill (broiler if you are American).

Chop the onion and the stalks and sauté them in the skillet in a little oil.

When the onion is translucent, spoon the vegetable mix into the mushrooms. Season to taste; in addition to salt and pepper I enjoy a light grating of nutmeg with mushrooms. Add the Napoli Sauce or tomatoes to each mushroom, adjusting to slightly overfill each cap.

Place the mushrooms in the skillet, add about a half-cup of water to the exposed area of the skillet to provide instant steam and also deglaze juices, then cover and cook over low heat for two or three minutes until the mushrooms have wilted. The stuffing will leak or spread a little and mix with the water to make a rich sauce.

Remove the lid and lightly cover the mushrooms with grated or sliced cheese. Sprinkle a little parmesan over the top. Place the skillet under the grill (broiler) until the cheese is bubbling and browning.

You can transfer it to a plate, but I usually eat it direct from the skillet on a trivet. That way I don't lose any of the sauce.

Oven Method.

Preheat oven to 200 C (390-400 F)

Prepare the mushrooms in the same way, but do not pre-cook anything. Assemble the mushroom caps, chopped onion and stalks, Napoli sauce and cheese in a suitable size ramekin or small baking dish. Add sufficient water to give a depth of about 6mm (1/4") in the ramekin after the mushrooms are placed in it.

Cook for approximately 15 minutes.
After the first time, you may need to adjust the time to suit your own oven.

I like this method for a fast breakfast because I can prepare it the night before and leave it in the oven pre-set to cook in the morning; ready when I wake. Allow a few minutes additional cooking time for the oven to reach the right temperature.

Nutrition Table

This is very approximate. The fat is from the olive oil and cheese, cut back on those if it worries you.

Calories	335
Kilojoules	1400
Protein	12 gm
Total Fat	25 gm
Carbohydrate	13 gm
Fibre	4.5 gm

Chili Crab

I developed this after I ate a wonderful Chili Crab in an apartment block cafeteria in Singapore on the way home from our first around-the-World trip in 2003. I kept experimenting until I came up with something with a similar flavour but without the sugar. As usual all portion sizes are very approximate.

Ingredients

For the sauce:
½ cup water
½ cup ketchup (I use Napoli Sauce) or 1/4 cup tomato paste
2 tablespoons soy sauce
1 teaspoon chilli flakes or 1 small chopped chilli (adjust to taste)
1 tablespoon vinegar
1 tablespoon splenda

For the wok or pan:
1 kg (2lbs) of fresh crab
1 tablespoon of peanut or olive oil
2 or 3 cloves of garlic, minced
Grated ginger to taste
1 chopped hot chilli to taste
1 sliced medium onion
1 teaspoon cornflour (cornstarch) or ¼ tsp guar gum
¼ cup water

Pre-cook the crab in boiling water. Divide the crab into appropriate portions, cracking legs and claws with the back of a heavy knife, and set aside. Mix the sauce ingredients and set it aside. Heat the oil in a wok or heavy pan and stir-fry the onion and chilli. Add the ginger and garlic and fry briefly. I often add some chopped celery or carrots or other greens at this stage as a variation.

Add the crab and stir-fry for two minutes then add the sauce and stir while heating for another five minutes or until the crab is heated through.

Mix the cornflour or guar gum and water and add to the pan. If you are using guar gum you will need a little practice to get the quantity right for consistency; if in doubt start with too little. Cook and stir until the sauce is thickened and ready to serve.

Serve as is or with basmati rice if the carbohydrates are OK for you. Supply damp towels for diners; they will need them. This is not a dish to serve to a food snob who won't use their fingers. Serves 2.

Nutrition Table

Calories	285
Kilojoules	920
Protein	35 gm
Total Fat	8 gm
Carbohydrate	18 gm

Made in the USA
Middletown, DE
14 September 2021